RUNNING
FREE

KATE ALLATT

and

ALISON STOKES

Published by Accent Press Ltd – 2011

Print ISBN 9781786157492
eBook ISBN 9781908006653

Cover design by Madamadari

To my amazing husband Mark, who saved my life,
and my equally amazing, yet remarkably resilient,
kids
– Indi, Harvey & The Woodster.
I love you so much.
Kate and Mum x

"Success is not final, failure is not fatal;
it's the courage to continue that counts."
Winston Churchill

Prologue

Sunday February 7 2010

I DON'T KNOW WHAT a migraine feels like. I've managed to live for thirty-nine years without ever having one. But if it makes you wish you could just take off your head and hand it over to someone else to look after until it stops yelling, then I guess the doctor at A&E must be right, that's what I've got.

Just four hours ago that same doctor sent me home with a packet of Co-codamol painkillers and told me to take it easy for a couple of days. I am trying my best to follow his advice which considering that I am mum to three active children isn't easy.

I've spent the afternoon lying in bed wishing the drugs would kick in and ease this relentless throb at the back of my head. I close my eyes and clutch the back of my neck, gently allowing my fingers to massage the base of my skull, wishing this agony would subside just long enough to let me drift off into a pain-free sleep. Please, just one hour of rest and I'll be OK.

Suddenly I hear 'MUM!' There's a brotherly war breaking out in the bathroom between Harvey, nine, and Woody, six. Woody's calling for backup. I try to block out their arguments knowing that my husband, Mark, who is down in the kitchen clearing up the remnants of Sunday lunch, will step in if it gets out of hand, as it usually does. But I can't ignore the noise. This headache is making me irritable. I get up from the bed and make my way to the bathroom.

'Harvey, if you don't leave your brother alone, you won't be going football training after school tomorrow,' I snap, causing another wave of nausea to wash over me. Mark hears my distress and comes to my rescue.

'You're stressing, sit down, I'll deal with them. Just calm down, and I'll make you a cup of Earl Grey tea,' he says, slightly irritated. Wrapping his arm around my shoulder, he guides me downstairs to the lounge, where I slump on the red leather sofa and cradle my head, which is throbbing so badly. This is the mother of all headaches. Our daughter India, eleven, has left the television on and gone upstairs to get her school bag ready for the morning. On the plasma screen there's a repeat of last week's *Dancing on Ice* where some soap star is twirling around like a pro. But I'm not really watching. I look at the clock on the TV screen. 6.09 p.m. I feel bad, really bad. Not just throbbing headache bad, but a sensation that I can't really describe. My body feels weak, like all the life is draining out of me. I start to panic.

'Mark, what's happening to me? I feel weird,' I shout to Mark who is just yards away in the kitchen. The words come out in a slur. 'Mmmeugh,' a stifled moan leaves my mouth and suddenly Mark is in front of me but his face is a blur. My entire body turns rigid and I panic as I slide off the sofa, landing on the floor in an inelegant heap. I feel Mark's arms around me as he tries to lift my dead weight and arrange my stiff limbs in to some semblance of comfort on the rug. I can only make out vague shapes and movement in the room, but I sense my husband's panic as he calls to our daughter, 'India, go and call Burt next door.'

2

Seconds pass, but I have no concept of time, just blind terror. I am no longer in control of my own body and it scares the shit out of me. Mark is still close, I can just about make out the whiteness of his T-shirt contrasting with the darkness of his hair.

'Please, help me. Don't leave me,' I beg inside my head.

I hear India's voice in the distance telling Mark that our neighbour is out and asking what's happening.

'Go and get Lise, just get anyone,' Mark responds, sending India to get help from our other neighbour, who also happens to be a nurse. The fear in his voice is rising as he holds me. Mark, my usually calm, sensible 'everything is black or white' kind of guy, is panicking. Right now, he can only see black.

'Kate, can you hear me? What's happening? Are you all right Kate?' Lise is here. I've no idea how long it's taken for her to arrive. I am hot, I want to reach out for something to fan myself with, but I can't move. My eyes are fixed wide open in fright like a rabbit caught in headlights. Now I can't even control my breathing, I struggle to gulp for air. I hear myself making desperate panting sounds. Lise sends India off to get a fan and shouts at Mark to call 999 quickly.

A paramedic is first to arrive. He listens to my heart and checks my blood pressure then gets on his radio to call for back-up, an ambulance for a 'lady in distress'. I wait. Mark and Lise are following the paramedic's advice and putting damp flannels on my forehead to keep me cool. But I still feel like I'm in the furnaces of hell. Maybe this is retribution for my lifestyle, running a home and business, ferrying the kids to their after-school clubs and activities and my own punishing fell-running regime. 'Is she having a fit?' Mark asks the paramedic.

3

'This is no fit,' is the stern response.

Minutes pass and we wait, all the time I feel weaker. The paramedic gets back on his radio. He's not taking any excuses. 'Send me any unit you can and send it now.' Even he seems to be panicking.

This is serious: Mark knows this is serious and I know it's serious. The paramedic tells Mark to go and get an overnight bag ready for me as I'm going to need it. I hear Mark's footsteps on the stairs and he returns with my running kit, silly sod. I know I love being out running on the fells, but running kit is the last thing I need at this moment.

Two men in green arrive and lift me onto a stretcher. As I'm wheeled out of my home, I think, where are the kids? I hope they don't see me like this. Then I wonder, am I wearing matching knickers and bra?

I feel a trickle running down the inside of my left thigh as I'm wheeled into the back of the ambulance. Oh great, now I've peed myself. How will I ever live with the embarrassment? Mark holds my hand as the sirens scream and I slip in and out of consciousness like someone is pressing the pause button on my life.

Chapter 1
Intensive Care Unit

Wednesday February 10 2010

'OH SHIT! WHAT'S HAPPENED here?' was my first thought when I regained consciousness. I was alive. But only just. I had been in a coma for three days. I could hear the noise of machines all around me in the intensive care unit. I was trussed up like a turkey. I had never seen so many tubes. They were up my nose, in my arms and worst of all was the monster tube stuffed in my mouth. I wanted to spit it out, but I couldn't move anything except my eye-lids. What I didn't realise was that the tube was also linked to the machine that was breathing for me. It was making me dribble, which is not a good look for anyone, especially a glamorous young mum like me. I don't feel glamorous right now, I feel scared.

I couldn't move yet my mind was functioning fine and working overtime. 'This is what it must feel like to be buried alive,' I thought to myself. Only this was worse because I could see life carrying on around me and had no way of being part of it. Doctors and nurses were huddled at the foot of my bed; they were mumbling about me. 'Hey, don't you know it's rude to talk about people when they're in the room,' I said. But of course my thoughts were silent. I couldn't speak and

I couldn't quite hear what they were saying about me, which was really annoying, but from the look on their faces I was someone to be pitied. As they walked away I heard laughter coming from the nurses' station. The drugs must have been making me paranoid because I thought they must be laughing at me. 'Come on, you guys, let me in on the joke. I've got a sense of humour. I could really do with something to cheer me up right now,' I was desperate for them to realise I was fun-loving Kate. I wanted to show them that underneath the tubes there was a nice, normal mother just like them, not some medical near-fatality. But they were gone in a blink. A nurse appeared with a clipboard and busied herself with one of the machines. She didn't even notice the tears of frustration running down my cheek. 'Please come and talk to me. I know I probably look like shit, but I won't bite.'

At least that headache had finally gone. The pain in the back of my head was the reason I was lying there so close to death. I later discovered that it hadn't been a migraine after all but a blood clot to the stem of my brain or, to put it bluntly, a massive stroke. I had been given a 50/50 chance of survival and for three days the doctors had been keeping me in a coma to give my brain a rest and the chance to recover. When I came round, I had been left 'locked in'. All my muscles – which controlled every movement in my body – were paralysed. Not only was I unable to sit up or move a finger, I could not even breathe or swallow for myself. I was completely helpless. Yet I was able to move my eyelids – I could open my eyes and watch everything in my field of vision. I could think for myself and understand everything that was going on around me. But did anyone know that I was alive inside my own paralysed body?

Then I realised I could also feel pain, my shoulder was really hurting after being stuck in the same position for three days. What I really wanted to do was roll over onto my side to give it a rest, but I couldn't.

The clock in front of my bed said 2.50 p.m. The kids would be finishing school soon. I panicked. Where was Mark? Was he waiting for them at the school gates? Time moves so slowly when you have no control over your body. All I could do was watch the minute hand on the clock tick forward and wish that someone would come over and tell me what was happening, spend some quality time with me. I've never been a clock-watcher. My life is too hectic with three kids, running my own business, a great circle of girlfriends and the fell-running, there are not usually enough hours in the day. But now all I could do was watch the clock and wait for someone, anyone, to take notice of me. After a day or two I realised that I couldn't even look forward to meal times. That too had been taken out of my hands and I was being fed through the tube up my nose. I couldn't feel it at the time, but I guessed that I must have a catheter tube draining off my urine at the other end.

Suddenly I have the awful feeling that I need a poo. Shit! I realised that I didn't even have control over my own bowels and I was wearing a nappy. I felt the sensation of something happening down below, like someone had put a cowpat in my knickers. I couldn't smell anything, but imagined that something unpleasant must be wafting across to the nurse's station opposite my bed. Surely a nurse will come to see me now.

If this was going to be my new life, I wanted it to end.

Chapter 2
Running, my Escape and my Amazing Friends

WHAT CAN I SAY about the life I had before it was taken away from me in such a sudden and undignified way? To anyone on the outside looking in, it must have appeared that I had it all. We were the typical middle-class family living the perfect suburban life.

Mark and I were newlyweds when we moved into our semi-detached 1930s home in the village of Dore thirteen years ago. We fell in love with the place and its rural charm. It was a good old-fashioned friendly Yorkshire community with thriving shops, pubs and a good primary school, just what we needed to start our family. More importantly, we had the beautiful south Yorkshire peak district on our doorstep and we made the most of it, spending all our spare time walking or mountain biking. We were married in Dore Church in 1998. One year later the first of our three children, India, was born. With Harvey and Woody our family was complete.

Mark and I both worked hard and poured our money into our home and family. Mark was a sales and marketing director for a company selling medical supplies, and I was just about to launch my own online digital marketing business, after years of working for other people. The children had their own busy social diaries: Girl Guides and dance lessons for India, football and rugby for Harvey and piano lessons and swimming for Woody. In our relationship I felt I was the passionate, creative one: the driving force. I would always set my goals above what most people would expect. I always wanted to push myself harder in my work and my personal life. Mark was more practical and grounded: my navigator. When I would go off on a flight of fancy he would try and rein me in. Between the two of us we made a good team.

Apart from my family, the two most important things in my life were my friends and my fitness. My closest friends were Alison, Anita and Jaqui, three other Dore village mums. We all had children of a similar age in the school and over the years our friendships developed through other common bonds. We were all 'superwomen' juggling the pressures of full-time jobs, running homes and still finding time to keep ourselves looking good and in shape. We were the Dore equivalent of the 'Desperate Housewives' – four thirty-something mums who walked a fine line between drama and domesticity on a daily basis.

Alison is my best and most loyal friend. She is the thoughtful and caring one. Married to a headmaster, Chris, I could trust her with my deepest secrets. Jaqui is the practical, efficient 'jolly hockey sticks' type. She has a high-powered government job and is married to a company director. Anita is the one all the blokes fancy. Half Indian and petite, she is a striking brunette with a dizzy blonde attitude, who runs her own pet-grooming business. Her husband, Bill, runs his own label and packaging company. In this mix I was the bloody-minded one, the tough nut, always making plans and getting results. When one of us was stressed, the others would help to ease the pressure. When one of the group was down, the others would arrange something as a treat. We enjoyed girlie nights in watching films, weekly book club meetings, fun weekends away being pampered at spas or soaking up the sun on Mediterranean beaches. Through our friendship, our husbands also became good mates too. Mark reckoned I could turn any event into a party and with Alison, Anita and Jaqui at my side, I generally did.

Our Saturday morning fell-running session was one of our regular get-togethers. For the past four years Jaqui and Anita and I would meet up and run. All weathers, all occasions, we would run. We'd take it in turns to plan a route, but each one was at least 12 miles. If it rained we would follow a path through the lower forests and if it snowed, as it occasionally did, we would just run that little bit faster. It always ended at a coffee shop. It was an all-weather, no-excuses session, our chance to catch up on the gossip as we ran. Our conversations covered four general themes for the week: how crap our husbands had been; how hectic work had been; how naughty the kids had been and the general village shenanigans of who had been spotted with someone they shouldn't have. After two hours and a cup of Earl Grey tea we would be set up for another week of stressful work and family life. When it was my turn to plan the route I would often lead the girls up to Froggatt Edge. At 20 miles it was one of our longer runs, but the views looking over the purple heather moors and the valleys below made it worthwhile. This snapshot of outstanding beauty was one that would stay in my mind when I was in hospital.

Our husbands all reckoned the running was pure fabrication after Mark once spotted us sitting outside a coffee shop in the village when we should have been halfway up a mountain. But our fitness spoke for itself.

Four days before my stroke I had been a guest on my local radio station, BBC Sheffield, talking about my big birthday challenge. June 3 2010 would be my fortieth birthday and I was determined to make it a year to remember. A couple of years earlier I had completed the Three Peaks Challenge. With a group of friends from work we had trekked to the top of the three highest peaks in England, Scotland and Wales in just twenty-four hours in aid of a local charity. For my birthday I wanted to push myself further and I was planning a series of challenges ending with a climb up Mount Kilimanjaro, Africa's highest mountain, in September. We were going to climb the most difficult western route. I was organising the event. Mark, Jaqui and I and five friends from the local rugby club were going. We had paid our deposits and booked our places for the challenge of a lifetime. We had just seven months to get into super-fit shape.

As part of my birthday challenge I had also signed the girls up for the Eyam Half Marathon in May, which is one of the toughest courses in Yorkshire, if not the whole of the UK. Over the course of thirteen and a half miles we would have to run 1200ft up on to the Yorkshire Moors, so I had convinced Anita that it would be a good idea to try an outdoor boot camp training session. We needed to push ourselves that bit harder and I thought that a two-hour session of military fitness was the wake-up call we needed.

At 7.45 a.m. on Saturday February 6, the day before my stroke, Anita picked me up and we drove out to Chatsworth House for the start of our new fitness regime. It was one of those perfect winter mornings, cold but crisp and we were excited at the thought of doing something a bit different. I had an extra buzz because for the first time in almost two weeks I had

11

woken up with a clear head, the annoying headache that I had been suffering from for the last fortnight had gone, and I felt on top of the world as our instructor ordered us to warm up in the clear, fresh, February morning air, while avoiding sheep poo in the grounds of the Duke of Devonshire's stately home.

'Kate, take it easy,' Anita warned me as I pushed my body to the limit with shuttle runs much faster than our instructor was expecting and twice the number of sit-ups and press-ups being asked of us. She knew that for me trotting around a field half-heartedly wasn't an option. I first introduced Anita to the Peak District's beautiful countryside when our children were still babes-in-arms. Our babies clocked up hundreds of miles in their early years as we lugged them miles and miles over the hills in all weathers in their baby rucksacks or pushed through the woods in their mud-splattered three-wheeler off-road prams. In return she introduced me to fell running. I had spent years road running and taking part in five and 10 kilometre charity runs like the Race for Life and had finished in a decent one hour thirty-eight minutes in the Sheffield half marathon, but I thought fell running would be easier on my ageing joints. Anita knows that when I do something I like to commit 200 per cent, some say it's the control freak in me, but I say it's determination. She also knew that two weeks earlier I had had a session with a personal trainer and ended up walking like I had been on a horse for weeks, so she was rightly concerned. On the way home we were buzzing from all the endorphins rushing through our bodies and made a pact that we would convince Jaqui to join us the following week.

When I got home, I ran myself a hot, bubbly bath while Mark went out on his usual weekend mountain bike ride. Harvey was at his football training, Woody

12

was swimming and India was in her bedroom listening to her iPod, so I had some well-deserved 'Me Time' and relaxed. Later that night Alison dropped her daughter Charlotte off for a sleep-over with India and while the girls were upstairs glued to Facebook the rest of the family sat down for our usual Saturday night around the telly, cuddled together on the sofa with a chicken tikka massala, pilau rice and onion bhajis from the village takeaway, and watched *Dancing on Ice* before having an early night.

Chapter 3
The Mother of All Headaches

THE FOLLOWING MORNING THE headache was back. My mouth was tingling too. I felt lousy and couldn't even blame it on the red wine from the night before as I had only managed a lightweight half a glass. I was due to go out for a run with Jaqui but texted her saying 'Don't feel like running. Headache's back.'

After breakfast Alison arrived to collect her daughter from a sleepover. I call Alison my partner in crime as we share the same love of life and silly sense of humour. She says I'm the only person tuned in to her wavelength. Never one to shy away from the truth, she said, 'You look dreadful.' I took that as an invitation to whinge about the headache that had been gnawing away at the bottom of my brain for the past two weeks. It wasn't so bad that it stopped me getting on with my daily routine, but it was annoying. It always seemed to be there, a real ache and a hindrance. The previous Saturday night my brother and his wife had come round for the evening with their kids and I had gone to bed early, which is very unusual for me. I thought it might have been caused by dehydration and had started to drink more water, but that only had the effect of making me pee more and did nothing to ease the pain.

After Alison had left, Mark, whom I suspected was

getting tired of my moaning, said, 'I've had enough of this; we're going to get it sorted.' Being a man, and therefore having a natural need to fix things, he rounded up the kids and drove to the local hospital. By the time we arrived the headache had developed from mildly annoying to something not being right. Mark dropped me and India off outside the entrance to the out-of-hours clinic and went to park the car with the boys. We walked up to the woman at the check-in desk. But as I tried to give her my name, my words came out in a slur and my vision started to blur.

'Is this the worst headache you've ever had in your life?' the nurse asked to which I replied, 'yes'. They tested my urine and although the nurse said they could find nothing obviously wrong she wasn't comfortable with the slurring incident and suggested I should go to the A&E department at the general hospital. I had three options: go immediately, go the following morning or book an appointment for the following day. 'We'll go now,' said Mark, who by this time had arrived from the car park with Harvey and Woody. The receptionist at the clinic called ahead to alert the A&E department and we drove across town to Sheffield Hallam Hospital.

An hour later I got to see the house officer in A&E. Some say you should avoid being seriously ill on a Sunday as that's when the consultants take their day of rest and the most junior of the junior doctors are on duty. By this time the Nurofen tablets that I'd taken earlier in the morning had started to work their magic and I didn't feel quite as bad; my speech and vision were OK. I explained what had happened in the clinic. 'Did you hear it?' the doctor asked Mark. He didn't. I sent Mark back out to the reception area to check on the children as in our panic we had left them alone in a busy A&E unit. Then the doctor asked me if anyone else had heard it, which they hadn't. At the time it struck me as an odd thing to ask. 'Do you have any worries in your life at the moment?' he asked. I explained how I was in the process of starting my own marketing company and was apprehensive about the responsibility of building a new client base and making enough money to pay the wages of my two new members of staff. He decided I was suffering from a migraine and sent me home with a couple of Co-codamol and instructions to 'keep an eye on it'.

With hindsight I know now that I should have challenged his diagnosis and argued that the nurse in the clinic was sufficiently worried about my slurring to send me for a second opinion. I should also have pointed out that, even though my blood pressure was normal, if he had looked at my medical notes he would have realised that 'normal' for me was actually low. But I did none of these things, I just went home, rested and waited for the blood clot in my brain stem to cut off the supply to my brain.

I don't remember much about the ambulance journey to A&E four hours later but I am told there was a manic flurry of activity as Mark called Alison to look after the children and I was rushed back into the same hospital, only this time I was wheeled in on a trolley with frantic paramedics at my side. The first person we passed was the doctor who had diagnosed a migraine earlier that afternoon. Mark later said he looked pretty pale when he saw us returning in emergency mode. I tried to shout something about having cramp in my leg. At this point Mark could see the terror in my eyes. I was a control freak who had no control over her own body. A mask was put over my face to sedate me as the doctors decided they needed to shut off a vein to my brain before taking me off for a scan. They warned Mark that 'something neurological was happening' but they didn't know what.

While my brain was being scanned Mark had the job of calling both our parents to break the uncertain news. He could not get a reply from my mum so rang my stepdad Dave and left an ominous massage. 'You've got to come urgently, something is happening to Kate.' They were at a friend's party in Bury, Bolton, and immediately made their excuses and drove to Sheffield. Next he called my dad, who was at home and also dashed directly to the hospital. His final call interrupted his parents' Sunday evening soiree. His mum and dad, both semi-retired with an active social life, were gearing up for a drinks party. When they got the call they put the dinner on the table, told their friends to help themselves, packed an overnight bag and set out on a lonely and nervous hundred-mile journey through the snow and fog.

Three hours later all sets of parents were gathered to hear the consultant deliver the news. I had suffered a right vertebral artery dissection and occlusion leading to an acute infarction in the pons or in layman's terms a massive clot in the main artery supplying blood to my brain. The CAT scan showed major damage and the prognosis was bleak. It was in such a delicate area that they could not operate, the only alternative was to use clot-busting drugs but they didn't know if it was too late. It was such a specialist area they needed to get advice from experts and some of the country's top neurologists were called at home.

This wasn't enough for Mark and my mum, they needed to know more. They needed definite answers and at that point there were no answers.

'It's pretty serious,' was all the doctor could say.

'We have got to get her through the next few hours. The next few hours are crucial.' Still at a loss to understand the magnitude of the situation, Mark pressed on.

'Does that mean she might not survive the night?'

'At best she has a 50/50 chance,' was the response.

As the minutes turned into hours, my family waited. It was too late for clot-busting drugs so the doctors decided that if I was to stand any chance of making it through the night they needed to shut down my body. I was moved into the Intensive Care Unit (ICU) and hooked up to machines that would keep me artificially alive. Mark and Mum stayed at my side looking for a faint glimmer of hope, but there was nothing: just the hissing of the respirator and the hypnotic beep of the heart monitor, but no movement. At 3 a.m. they were told to go home. There was nothing more they could do. They could only wait. As they walked out to the car the floodgates opened and they broke down in a tearful embrace as the critical nature of my predicament hit them – they might never see me alive again. That night my mum prayed and Mark slept: the rest of an exhausted powerless man.

Chapter 4
Eight out of Ten is Bad

WHILE I LAY IN a coma it was school as normal for my children. Mark decided they needed some sort of stability in their lives, as much for his sanity as their protection. He knew that if he allowed himself to stop and dwell on the situation for even a second, he would fall apart. He also knew that I had poured all my attention and affection into our children and if he let that go to waste I would come back and haunt him. Besides what could he honestly tell the children when he did not know what was happening himself?

They had gone to bed the previous night knowing I was ill and woke up to find an empty space in the kitchen where I would usually be filling their cereal bowls and nagging them to hurry up. Over breakfast Mark explained that Mummy was very poorly in hospital and that everything was to carry on as normal. 'I'll take you to school and when you come home everything will be OK.' It was stretching the truth of course, but they seemed to accept it.

The school run that morning was hard for both Mark and Alison. Alison could not make eye contact or speak to any of the other mothers for fear of breaking down. When she had said goodbye to Mark in the early hours of the morning when he had got home from the hospital there was only half a chance I might survive. She could not talk to him for fear of what the news might be. Anita, always the intuitive one, sensed something had happened and when Alison broke the bad news they agreed to keep it to themselves until there was more information to share. In the days that followed, as news of my illness spread throughout the village, the school run became even more difficult as more and more mums avoided Mark. You'd think he was the one with some horrible illness. Everybody was shocked but nobody knew what to say. They all had questions but being a polite, middle-class village no one wanted to be the first to upset him. But my mum and friends helped him through the very difficult first couple of days.

After the school run my family gathered in the visitors' room at the ICU for a briefing with the doctors and care staff. It was an awkward and silent meeting as from the medics' point of view there really was very little more they could say. I had survived the night, which was a bonus, but the next aim was to get me through to the end of the week. Mark needed to understand how bleak the prognosis was, asking, 'On a scale of nought to ten, with ten being dead, how bad is Kate?' He was expecting a middling reply of five but the answer came back as eight. That's when it really hit home how close to death I was. Mum was horrified, both by the matter-of-fact way that Mark had put my life on a sliding scale and also at the bleakness of the response. She needed to have a glimmer of hope to restore the natural balance of motherhood that says your children should outlive you. One of the doctors, an Irishman, must have noticed the stunned expression on Mum's face and explained that the brain is a remarkable thing, and that he had seen a case like mine where there had been progress, and that if progress was to happen then, once it started, it was usually quick, with the patient making a near-normal recovery. But this glimmer of hope was clouded by his overriding comment, that I was very poorly indeed, and that many people with a severe brain-stem injury like mine did not make a good recovery. The likelihood was that if I did live I would be dependent for the rest of my life.

'It's not good,' said Mark, voicing everyone's inner thought. The doctors nodded in agreement.

In the days that followed Mark adopted the approach: 'Life ain't good but we've got to get on with it.' At work he told his immediate boss but said nothing to his other colleagues as he didn't want to answer any difficult questions. With the help from my mum and his parents, he began a daily routine of work, hospital and bed. Once the children were in bed at 8.30 Mark would also go to bed and sleep. He could not allow himself to sit down and think; he knew that if he did he would slip over the edge into a dark place from which he might never be able to return. Mark later told me that for months after my stroke he was unable to bring himself to sit in our lounge, where the drama had started, it made him feel too lonely.

It's amazing that in the most desperate of times the simplest things can make you laugh. And for Mark and my family it was a lost fish pie and a Friday night out with the lads.

As soon as the word of my illness spread, the Dore community sprang into action. There was little they could do in terms of hospital visits, so they baked comfort food for all the family, for which Mark was very grateful. The ladies of the church rallied round and set up a cooking rota. Considering we had not set foot in the church since our wedding almost twelve years earlier, with the exception of the annual Christmas Eve carol concert, it was a particularly kind gesture. Every day there would be another dish waiting on the doorstep: hearty casseroles, pots of chilli con carne, saucepans of Bolognese. But the one that never arrived was the fish pie. My stepdad Dave was particularly looking forward to the promise of his favourite pie. That evening when they arrived home from the hospital there was no fish pie. They asked around but no one had seen it. Not wanting to seem ungrateful they sent their thanks back to the cook before they had even found it. The mystery was unravelled a couple of days later when one of the kids moved a school bag from the porch and hiding underneath was the missing fish pie.

Soon afterwards a group of the Dore husbands and Mark's mountain-biking friends invited him to the pub to unwind with a Friday night beer. Mark got more than he bargained for when he said, 'I've been so busy, I've not even had time for a wank!' To which one of the group said, 'if I can do anything to help, please ask.' He didn't realise his gaffe and Mark didn't take him up on the offer but they have all laughed about it since!

Chapter 5
Alive Inside

COMING OUT OF THE coma, I was aware of everything going on around me as the doctors and nurses battled to save lives. Over the hissing of the ventilators and the beeping of the heart monitors, I could hear the muffled voices of the staff as they discussed the bleak prognoses of the other patients. But I could do nothing to make them understand that I was alive and listening.

I could feel every ache in my body and each one seemed to be magnified. The pain in my shoulder wouldn't go away and nothing I could do would ease it. Propped up with two pillows under my arms and tubes in every orifice, I felt as if I was the victim of some bizarre torture ritual.

I kept my eyes fixed on that damned clock, it was all I could do. Curiously, although I was completely paralysed I could open and close my eyelids at will. My tears were a mixture of voluntary and involuntary reactions born out of sadness, frustration and the need to attract attention. Blinking was the only thing I had control over, getting someone to realise it, however, was completely out of my control and led to more tears.

At 4.17 p.m. a middle-aged nurse with a bun and a blonde auxiliary nurse appeared at the side of my bed. They were chatting amongst themselves and looking over me, not at me. The older of the nurses had a syringe in her hand and injected painkillers into a cannula inserted in the back of my right hand. She said nothing, all the time avoiding eye contact, but I could feel the coolness of the drugs slipping into my blood stream. Then they rolled me over from my back onto my left side. It was the first time I was aware of what was a four-hourly ritual to stop me developing bedsores. Tears started to roll down my cheek. I tried to blink them away but they trickled into my mouth. I could not understand why the nurses were not talking to me. I was still desperate to be told what was happening. I wanted so much for them to see through the tubes and charts to the person lying inside the paralysed shell. I imagined that in a different life, these women who had found their vocation saving lives, would be the sort of independent, motivated women who I would be happy to call my friends, if only given half a chance. Later I learned that they thought I was brain-dead and my tears were my way of grieving for my old life.

'Smells like someone needs changing,' the older nurse mutters to her colleague as they get a whiff of the contents of my nappy. Drawing the curtains around my bed, I realise it's time for the first of many indignities. As they stripped me and rolled me from one side to the other, wiping my bottom and bundling the dirty pads into a nappy bag, I tried to block out the embarrassment. I closed my eyes. In my mind I was running over the hills, imagining the sensation of fresh morning mountain air in my lungs.

Job done, the nurses move off to the next bed, their voices fading into the background beneath the whirring and beeping of the machines. Once again I was left counting the minutes. 'Where is Mark?' I wonder. 'Does he know I'm alive?' 'Why won't anyone talk to me?'

An hour passed, but in this nether-world of drugs and death it seems like an eternity. Then I saw a familiar face at the end of my bed.

'God you gave us a scare,' Mark says, trying to sound upbeat and hide his fear when faced by the wreckage of his wife. Mark has never known me to be ill – apart from the time I broke my right arm playing rugby at college. Even when I had a Caesarean section to give birth to Woody I was back on my feet and in the gym within three days. To see me lying in a coma for the past three days has been a massive shock. Although my eyes are slightly open, and there's a flicker of hope, conversation is very much one way.

I am so relieved to see him. Avoiding all the tubes, Mark sits down by the bed and gives me a hug. I try to move my hand to clasp his fingers. Nothing. I try to move my foot. Nothing. I don't know what has happened to me. Involuntary tears roll down my face and I have no way of hiding them as Mark talks about his day at work and home and holds back his own tears.

'Your mum is at home, looking after the kids. Kate, you have to get better, you know I can't live with your mother 24/7,' he says trying to make light of the dark situation. I want to tell him I'm alive, but I have no way of communicating, Mark always used to tell me that my eyes could speak more than words. He always joked that when he came home from work he knew if he was in trouble, just by looking at my eyes. Now I can only stare hoping he will realise I am trying to connect with him. I want to ask him if he has paid the subscriptions for Woody's Beavers group. I want to know if India, Harvey and Woody saw me being wheeled away in an ambulance and if they are as frightened as I am.

I fix my eyes on Mark as he talks, but his expression

seems vague. I wonder if the doctors have told him the truth. Does he know I am going to die? Is this his last goodbye? I am scared he will look at me in this crippled state and walk away. As Mark talks, a thought pops into my head and makes my eyes smile. 'This is the first time you've been able to get the upper hand in a conversation with me, so enjoy it.' I watch his lips move, wanting so much to take his face in my hands and kiss him hard. My memory drifts back to the night we met in Sheffield Rugby Club in February 1990.

I was nineteen and in my first year at Sheffield University, determined to enjoy the student life. I had set out to get involved with all the clubs I could, or at least the ones that liked a laugh. I joined the women's rugby team, not because I loved the thrill of a good ruck but more because those girls knew how to party after a game. Similarly I joined the Irish Society because I heard the 'craic' was good.

Mark was twenty-three and played for Sheffield Rugby Club's first team. He was propping up the bar with his rugby mates and about to down his seventh pint of snakebite (lager and cider mixed) with blackcurrant when he announced, 'Next girl through the door I'm going to ask to dance.' In I walked, followed by my friends. It was late in the evening, I was going through a dry spell after having met loads of boys in the first term and so I was up for a laugh. The DJ played the opening riff of 'Don't Bang The Drum' by The Waterboys and we didn't so much dance as side-step, my pint sloshing over the dance floor as we staggered around in time to the music in our heads, not to the tune that was playing. We laughed and I teased him that his tie was standing up on its own. He was full of beer and I was pretty drunk too. When the music ended we went back to the bar and I challenged him to a drinking contest. Last one to down a pint of snakebite and blackcurrant would buy the next round. He must have looked at me, this nine-stone, lanky teenager and thought there was no competition, but he didn't realise this was my party piece and I had become quite skilled in downing cider, having learnt to hustle men for drinks during my sixth-form years. With all his macho rugby mates cheering him on, I narrowly beat him. Mark never lived the incident down. Maybe at this point he should've made his excuses and left, but instead he offered to walk me home to the student village.

Two weeks passed before I heard from Mark again. After our drunken night at the rugby club we had said goodnight without swapping names or addresses, those were the days before mobile phones. Mark had a vague idea that I lived in a village of hundreds of student rooms but I had no idea where he lived, and anyway had no intention of chasing him. Luckily Mark took the initiative and returned to the student village, knocking on random doors until he found where I lived and left a message with a neighbour. We had our first date at a local pub. In his mind he was chasing the girl with the long dark hair and the 'lovely bum' he had met at the rugby club. When we actually met I arrived looking like an extra from the Hair Bear Bunch as I had recently had one of those awful perms that were fashionable in those days, and wasn't looking my best. Again Mark had the chance to make his excuses and escape, but he didn't, which I thought was a good sign. We spent the night chatting and learning more about each other. I found out that Mark worked as a metallurgist, one of those brainy scientific types who worked with metal at one of the Sheffield steelworks and shared a house in the city with his mate. Underneath the bizarre haircut, Mark discovered that I had been a nanny in America, now back home in Sheffield and studying business with ambitions to one day run my own nanny agency. Apart from our love of rugby and the ability to down pints of snakebite in record time, we had common interests in outdoor activities like mountain biking, walking and skiing. At the end of the evening Mark asked me if I wanted half a bed or half a taxi fare home, cheapskate! That made me like him even more. He respected my independence and didn't assume that I would want to jump into bed with him. As it happened, I didn't choose between the half bed or the taxi, I fell asleep on Mark's bathroom floor.

Over the next five years our relationship grew as friends and lovers. We were comfortable in one another's company and could talk for hours about any old nonsense. Before I met Mark I had no confidence with boys. I had two brothers and a half sister, Abi, who was 14 years younger. My brother Paul was two years older, while Tim was a year younger, and I was the tomboy sandwiched in the middle, so I grew up thinking boys were annoying. At school I was never the pretty one or the trendy one; I was Kate the country bumpkin. Coming from out-of-town, working-class Macclesfield, my friends and I were nicknamed 'the sheep shaggers' at school by the trendy city kids. Although on the outside I was bursting with bravado and cockiness when Mark and I met, inside I was deeply insecure. I had been dumped by my two previous serious boyfriends and my self-esteem was at an all-time low. At first I put up a barrier and wouldn't allow Mark to get too close for fear of being hurt again, but Mark seemed to like me. As the months stretched into years our relationship became more settled.

The competitive streak that started with the cider drinking continued throughout our relationship in a friendly, almost sibling-like, rivalry. We would go out walking and I would always walk faster and further. One day while walking in the Peak District in the winter we found a frozen pond and I punched a hole in the ice. Dipping my bare hand in I challenged Mark, 'Bet you can't do this?' He plunged his hand into the sub-zero, icy water close to mine. With our eyes locked, hands barely touching, we stood there shivering, neither one prepared to give in. Eventually I nearly got frostbite but I won. Like two little kids we would always be daring one another to do dafter, and sometimes more dangerous, things like jumping in reservoirs. For my twenty-first birthday we bought mountain bikes and took them off to France for a three-week camping holiday in the back of Mark's VW Polo. I remember we drove 2,500 miles in the scorching heat. When we got the bikes out, Mark would race off and I would pedal like hell to catch up with him. Another time we went skiing in Switzerland and spent all day, every day, on the slopes until we were too exhausted to do anything else. We were in love but, more importantly, we were best mates.

Now when I looked at Mark I could see the fear in his eyes. There was no longer any competition between us. He could walk, talk, breathe, eat, sleep and shit. I could do nothing. Every day Mark would visit and sit beside me for hours. He later said that it was sometimes like 'talking to a piece of wood' yet he always managed to maintain a jokey and flippant façade. Some days his optimism would cheer me up, but on the days when I was feeling sorry for myself, I would be shouting inside, 'Sod off and leave me alone.' Occasionally Mark would bring in a camera and take photos of me. At the time I hated it as I really wasn't looking my best and felt it was an invasion.

When he left the ward, I found out later, Mark would break down in tears because of the cruel nature of my injuries. I would also weep for the woman I used to be. My mind would go back to the early days of our relationship when we split up after five years because he wasn't ready for marriage and kids and I was. My mum was only eighteen when she had my brother and my body clock was ticking. Now we had taken our vows 'in sickness and in health'; we had three beautiful children, yet I had nothing to offer Mark, just a future of caring for me. I would think, when are you going to get fed up of this one-way conversation and leave me? My insecurities linked back to those of my own childhood and would run riot. I would think about the ten-year-old Kate who was hurt when her mother walked out on her family and set up a new life with Dave. In reality Mark had never shown anything but loyalty and support, apart from one indiscretion early on in our relationship when we were still young, but inside there was a nagging voice that wouldn't shut up. Lying in the ICU my paranoia ran riot.

Chapter 6
The Indignity of it All

I WAS PUMPED SO full of drugs that I have very little recollection of those early days in the ICU, but the overriding feeling was one of fright and frustration. Fear that no one was telling me what was going on and frustration from being reduced from being an independent, active woman to a needy hospital patient totally dependent on the whims, seemingly, of the overworked ICU staff.

During this time I began to realise that the doctors and nurses in the ICU are efficient and skilled when it comes to monitoring machines, administering live-saving drugs and keeping patients artificially alive, but they don't have much of a bedside manner. I guess when you mostly deal with people who are comatose or brain-dead you don't get much chance to brush up on your social skills.

Day after day they busied themselves with filling in charts, recording data and keeping me alive, but no one realised that I was taking in everything they were saying. They had made the assumption that I was brain-dead and was unable to comprehend anything that was happening around me. On a ward where people were dying or being brought back from the brink on a daily basis, being locked in sometimes felt worse than being dead.

For a start I was in constant pain. Every part of my body seemed to ache, cramp would wash over my legs, arms and neck in waves of agony. My bum was sore from the bed, my feet were hot and uncomfortable from the splints holding them straight. Lying there, I had all the time in the world to dwell on my aches and pains. I would feel the cramp starting in my foot and brace myself for the searing pain as it shot up my leg. When I was at home I would sometimes wake Mark up in the middle of the night, hopping around the room to ease a sudden bout of cramp, but in the ICU I was powerless. I would desperately try to attract the nurses' attention, following them around the room with my eyes, imploring them to notice the agony I was in.

'Please help me. Please, it's hurting. Aaaghh!' I would scream in my head as another spasm rushed through my body. But my silent cries and begging eyes went unnoticed, bringing tears of frustration as well as pain.

'If death means an end to all this agony, bring it on,' I would think to myself at my lowest point as I contemplated the least horrible way I could shuffle off this mortal coil. To me the idea that I could be injected with an overdose of drugs, like an animal being put out of its misery, seemed wrong. In my head I played out the imaginary scene with a nurse or doctor at my side to give the lethal dose. That was no good, I had a notion I wanted to die on my terms. I wanted someone I loved to be the one to end my miserable life. I wanted Mark to be the one with me when I took my last breath. I had no means of communicating this wish to him, but deep inside I wished he would put a pillow over my head. I was in no position to struggle, I could just drift off into a pain-free sleep. My family and friends would be better off without me in this state. They would grieve for me, but in time they would come to terms with their loss, get on with their lives and remember me as the woman I had been: lively and full of energy.

The tiredness added to these feeling of depression. Ever since I had come out of the coma I had been unable to sleep. The nights were never-ending and the days were a constant battle to stay awake in the vain hope of getting a decent night's sleep. The incessant, mechanical hiss of the machines should have been hypnotic, but the sound just annoyed me. On top of this there was one patient, an elderly man with dementia, who would shout and lash out at the nurses. By day his raised voice was upsetting but in the silence of the night his bellows were amplified and added to my vulnerability. It upset me to hear the way he was speaking to the nurses and I worried that he might turn on me, even though realistically there was no way he could climb over the cot-sides of his bed.

One night I was in so much pain, I closed my eyes and drifted off for what I thought was the last time. I felt as if I was on the edge of a chasm, but there was nothing beyond it. I have never been a particularly religious person and had no concept of what the after-life would bring. But I had heard stories of bright lights and tunnels leading to peace. For me there was no light, no one to guide me to the other side, just darkness. When I woke up it had just been wishful thinking. I was still in pain and the idea that there was no higher being on the other side just made me feel more lonely and depressed.

In my drug-addled paranoid state I took a dislike to one of the nurses, an older woman whose lack of eye contact and empathy I took as a sign that she thought I would be better off dead when probably all she was concerned about was keeping me alive. There was a nurse with a Stoke accent who was also always busy tending to the machines but at least I felt she had a kindly manner as she checked the charts at the foot of my bed and went about her business. Then there was a pretty young nurse, who would spend time talking to me and was caring beyond her eighteen years.

Every morning the doctors carried out their rounds and stopped at the bottom of my bed. I could not quite hear what they were saying above the muffled noises of the machines, but I thought they were discussing whether I was worth keeping alive and I was terrified they would come to the conclusion that I was not worth the effort and that the bed could be used for a more deserving case.

One of the things that scared the hell out of me at this time was that the life support machine seemed to develop a will of its own. The tube that was pumping oxygen into my body would pop off without warning. This happened at least four or five times a week and I would be forced to lie there listening as the oxygen that was destined for my lungs hissed out into the air, knowing that I was being starved of my lifeline. Often it took no more than ten seconds for the nurses to be alerted to the problem and push the tube back on. But in those seconds I was reminded how fragile my life was and how I really was in the hands of the medical team and machines.

During those early days in the ICU two other patients died. One was an elderly man with a serious chest infection, the other was a forty-year-old father of two who had suffered a massive heart attack. Before the younger man died I overheard the doctors and senior nurses talking with his family. They were discussing the withdrawal of his care and feeding as he was being kept alive artificially. A couple of days later he was gone and his family was devastated. I lay there and listened as his family gathered around his body and cried. He was a young parent like me and this incident affected me greatly. I had heard of cases where people who were in a persistent vegetative state had had their care withdrawn and were allowed to die. At this early stage I believed that, as none of the medical staff or my family had realised my mind was working, they might decide to withdraw my food too and allow me to pass away. I panicked. What if the doctors were having a similar conversation with my family? Given the hard choice of allowing me to live as a 'vegetable' or pulling the plug, what would they opt for? Mark had always said that if anything drastic happened to him he would never want to be kept alive 'unable to wipe his own arse'. I had been more philosophical during these what-if conversations and said I could not decide. I replayed those conversations over and over in my mind, feeling more and more vulnerable with every hypothetical outcome. Knowing how much I loved life and my independence and how important my health and fitness was to me, what if my next-of-kin thought that the best outcome for me would be death? Given the choice would my family agree to switch off the life support without ever realising my mind was working? Tears of terror rolled down my cheek as I wondered how I could convince my family I was alive inside and capable of making my own life-or-death decisions.

That night I had a vivid dream that the man in the bed next to mine was being killed. To this day I am still not sure whether I was awake or sleeping when it happened, but it is one of the more lasting and disturbing memories I have of the ICU. In my dream the doctors were giving the patient an electric shock instead of a chest massage. Like me, the man was convinced they wanted him dead and he cried out, 'I'm not worth keeping.' On another occasion, I dreamed that at night a nurse switched my drip for graphite, designed to slowly reduce my heart rate to a stop. I imagined it so vividly, and it was deeply traumatising that in my dream I was powerless to stop my impending death.

But the drugs did do funny things to my imagination. I remember having another realistic dream where I thought I was Patrick Duffy in the TV series *The Man From Atlantis*. When I was a teenager in the eighties I, like many teenager girls, had a massive crush on Patrick Duffy who went on to play Bobby Ewing in *Dallas*. Lying in bed I imagined that I had webbed feet like the Man from Atlantis and that I would be able to swim away or that I would return from the death bed like Bobby Ewing in the famous *Dallas* shower scene.

Unfortunately for me my feet weren't webbed, they were strapped into hideous, uncomfortable leg braces. Even though the doctors had already decided that, if I lived, I would never walk again, they thought they would play safe and strap my legs into metal frames. This had the effect of preventing my feet from twisting like tree roots should I ever get out of bed. It also made them unbearably hot and gave me cramp in my legs. One thing amazingly I found I could do was cry at will. Sometimes I would cry to attract the nurses' attention to the pain, but it rarely worked.

I hated the tube in my mouth. I dribbled relentlessly and it made it impossible to sleep at night. Yet the doctors said I was 'tube tolerant'. 'Is that a good thing?' Mark asked at the time only to be told no as it showed I had lost gag reflex. I later learned that insomnia can be one of the many side-effects of locked-in syndrome. It didn't help that the nursing night staff often used the empty bay next to my bed as a meeting place. In the distance I could hear them laughing and chatting. I couldn't hear what they were saying but I could sense they were having fun. I was desperate to be included. I was so desperate for the nurses to treat me like I was a real person – not some fragile pain in the arse who was interrupting their daily routine.

At 8 every morning two nurses would come to my bed with a bowl of water and a flannel and close the curtains around my bed. 'How are we this morning?' they would say in a patronising tone as if they were talking to a toddler. I would blink hard, my way of saying 'sod off and leave me alone' but it went unnoticed as they continued to strip me and roll me from one side to the other, rubbing soap and water into every intimate nook and cranny. The first time when they changed my dirty nappy was the worst, but it never got easier. Each time I closed my eyes and tried to shut out the indignity. The twenty-minute routine would end with me being smothered in moisturiser and dressed in a new gown. Some gowns were old and soft, others were new and stiff with starch. I looked forward to getting an old one as they were more comfortable. As the days dragged on I grew to enjoy this perverse pampering session. I wouldn't normally have enough time to spend slapping on lotions and potions in the morning while I was rushing to get three kids ready for school. The mums at the school even had a collection and bought me a tub of expensive Clarins moisturiser, which was nice even if it was partly wasted on someone who had no sense of smell.

Another of the excruciatingly embarrassing indignities that I had to deal with around this time was the start of my 'monthlies', as the ward sister described it. My mum was asked to bring in some night-time sanitary pads which were attached to my nappy. I would later refer to them as my 'crash-mats' and they became another sign of an embarrassing bodily function that I was unable to control.

After my daily bathing routine, my physiotherapist, a caring New Zealander who wore high-waistbanded trousers like Simon Cowell, would hoist me out of bed like a sack of spuds and manoeuvre my limbs to keep my muscles active. After an exhausting morning I quite often fell asleep in the afternoon while watching the clock and waiting for my first visitors.

Chapter 7
We've Had Our Differences but my Mum's Great

MY MUM NEVER CRIES. She's like me, or maybe I'm like her. All through my childhood I never saw my mother cry. She never really showed any sign of emotion. It wasn't that she didn't love her kids, but she came from that post-war generation of stoic mums who just put on a brave front and got on with life. If she was upset she would hide away and cry, never wanting to show her weakness. I've inherited that from my mum, in times of trouble and stress I too run away and hide and bounce back when I'm stronger and ready to face the world.

When I saw my mum crying for the first time, it reinforced the fact I was in a bad way. Of course Mum didn't know I could see her tears and register her pain or she wouldn't have shown this sign of weakness. 'Please, Mum, tell me what's wrong with me?' I wanted to beg her.

Since the night of the stroke she had kept a daily vigil at my bedside. She had watched helplessly as my breathing had lurched up and down. When the doctors thought my breathing was getting stronger they would turn the ventilator down a notch, minutes later my breath would take a nosedive and they had to rush over and turn it back up. Watching all this drama was not good for her. Even worse was the wait to be allowed on to the ICU ward. Mum hates hospitals at the best of times and having to gather together with all the other visitors in a grim room outside and wait for clearance was sheer hell for her. Depending on how busy the staff were, it could take ages. Mum would stand in front of the window, peering into the gloomy world of death and artificial respiration, take a deep breath and count down from ten before entering. She later told me that those visits were the hardest thing she ever had to do. I would lie there, following her with my eyes, as she tidied my locker and rearranged the lotions and potions. It was her way of showing her love when words failed her as they often did. When my locker, which was full of useless things I had no need for, like tea bags and toothpaste and clean cotton pyjamas, was as neat as it could be, Mum would start tidying me. She'd massage my twisted feet and try to rearrange them into a position that looked half-normal. On the occasions when our eyes met and I would try to hold her gaze long enough to make her understand I was alive, I looked at the door as if to say, 'Take me home, please Mum' but it seemed futile. She'd smile and look away. I wondered how long it would take before Mum noticed it was no coincidence the way my eyes were following her around the room.

Sometimes Mum would break the silent monotony of these visits by bringing her husband Dave for back-up. Several years younger than Mum, Dave has been like a surrogate dad to me for almost 30 years. When I was younger he never tried to impose his values on his step-family but earned our trust through mutual respect. Since the age of 10, Dave has been a constant in my life, mending broken toys and broken hearts, handing out advice and money in my times of need.

Each time I see Dave I want to say, 'Hey, Dave,

how's your shed?' He spends hours in his retreat at the bottom of the garden, Mum jokes that his wood-turning tools get more attention than her. I watch as he moves his face close to mine as if to kiss me. 'I'm sorry, Kate, but I can't fix this,' he whispers, choking back the emotion. I feel the tears flow again and Dave wipes them away, oblivious to the fact that I am understanding everything he says.

Throughout those early days in the ICU when my prognosis was bleak, my mum was buoyed by the words of the Irish consultant who had explained that the pathways in my brain which controlled all my movements were no longer functioning. He had said that the brain sometimes has the ability to open up new pathways and this gave Mum hope. She would stare at me for hours looking for the faintest twitch or flicker of movement, which she took to be a positive step on the brain's path to recovery.

'You know what, our Kate?' she whispered, her broad accent – a mix of Welsh and Cheshire with a hint of Scouse – wavering with emotion. 'You've always been a strident one. If there are new paths in your brain, you can find them,' she would say as she massaged my feet with expensive Chanel moisturiser.

Listening to Mum's soothing tone, I drifted back in my head to a time when she wasn't so delicate. 'You are not going there!?' Mum shouted down the phone when I called to tell her I had booked a one-way ticket to Bangkok.

It was March 1995 and my relationship with Mark had hit a rocky patch after five years. A girl I thought was a friend turned out to be a jealous boyfriend snatcher. When I discovered they had been having an affair. I knew I had to run away. A letter arrived from Diana, one of my oldest friends from Catholic

41

secondary school, inviting me to stay with her, and I saw my chance to escape and patch my broken heart. I booked a flight to Bangkok, handed in my notice at the government office where I worked and packed a bag. I said nothing to Mark until I was ready to go; I had made up my mind to leave. I was hurting and, like a wounded animal, I wanted to take myself away from the pain to gather my strength. Mum told me I was mad to just take off. I was twenty-four years old and she thought I had finally grown up and settled down but here I was heading off to Thailand like some gap-year teenager. She thought I should go back home to her, sort out my differences with Mark and move on with my life.

I thought a couple of months of escapism, sun, sea and cheap booze in Thailand was a better idea than a damp spring in Macclesfield.

As I was getting ready to leave for the airport I called Mark to tell him I was going to Bangkok on a one-way ticket. He rushed home from work to convince me to stay. But if there was one thing I had shown him in our five years together it was that I was a stubborn sod and if I set my mind on something then nothing would stand in my way. I had £200 in my pocket, but I returned nine months later with £2000 and a head full of wild memories

There's a reason they call the capital city of Thailand backpackers' paradise. With its heady mixture of cheap booze, drugs on demand and sex for sale, and its location at the gateway to Australasia, it's a popular stop-off for young Europeans, American and Australians on their travels around the world. Diana had been there for several months working as a part-time teacher to a wealthy Thai family. The husband was the son of the owners of one of Thailand's leading pharmaceutical companies. We nicknamed him 'Petch the Letch' because of his hobby of taking photos of his English employees. His wife had one of the top jobs in education. They had two children, aged four and eighteen months, and employed Diana as a part-time teacher to their eldest who had failed an entry exam. The family had four other nannies and wanted a full-time English governess, just like Anna and the King of Siam. When I arrived with my American nanny qualifications on my CV they offered me the job and I took it straight away. They even asked me how much I wanted to earn. Our plan was to spend four months in Bangkok then move on to Australia.

For those four months I went mad. We spent our free weekends at Petch's holiday home by the sea in Hua Hin. Diana and I flew across to the island of Koh Samui for a two-week holiday where we swam in the clear blue waters and had massages on the beach. We took the night train over the border to Laos, where I smoked 'herbal cigarettes' with complete strangers. We travelled to Malaysia in search of adventure. And we risked our lives by getting tattoos on the Khao San Road. In his bestselling book *The Beach* Alex Garland famously described Khao San Road as 'the centre of the backpacking universe'. It was a place where the vibe was chilled and anything did go – including health and safety. We were celebrating my twenty-fifth birthday and thought it would be a good idea to have a cute creature inked onto our hips. The backstreet tattoo artist was a fat pig of a man, who advertised his skills on a real live pig that was completely covered in tattoos and stood in the shop. The owner had so many piercings in his ears he looked like an over-used dartboard. He wore a sweat-stained vest and held a rolled-up cigarette in his dirty fingers. 'You wait twenty minutes so bacteria on needle die,' he said. Sounded fair enough. We had taken just ten minutes to choose our designs, a butterfly for me and a ladybird for Diana, but didn't mind waiting an extra ten minutes to ensure a semi-sterile needle. Looking back to 1995 when the AIDS virus was a major killer and was transmitted through dirty needles, the butterfly tattoo could have been the death of me. Luckily it wasn't.

When our four months in Thailand was up we gave Petch and his wife our notice and jetted off to Australia for the final leg of our adventure. For the first few weeks we travelled around the east coast on a Greyhound bus, stopping off at surfers' paradise Byron's Bay, the Gold Coast and Cape Tribulation in the north-east. Arriving in Sydney, Diana and I finally went our separate ways. She wanted to get the bus to Ayers Rock and I wanted to stay in Sydney. I booked myself into a sixteen-dollar-a-night hostel and stayed two weeks until my money ran out. I was washing car windows at traffic lights to make money, but it wasn't enough. I was down to my last few dollars and desperate for a job when I picked up a copy of the *Sydney Herald.* 'Nanny wanted for three weeks.' It was the ideal job, so I called the number only to discover that I was too late, they had already had loads of applications. 'But you have to see me,' I persisted. 'I am an English governess and an au pair in the US.' Eventually the woman on the other end of the phone gave in and agreed to see me at 3 p.m. I arrived at 2 p.m. and spent the next hour making friends with her three boys. We played basketball and cards and by the time of my interview, the job was as good as mine. I was put on trial to babysit for the night. So I slept over and next morning as we sat around the coffee table they offered me the job. I was thrilled, but there was just one problem. The couple wanted a nanny while they went off to Europe for three weeks, but they were not due to leave for another two weeks. I needed the job now. I had enough money for one more night at the hostel but if I couldn't find more work I'd have to face the shame of calling Mum and asking for money for a flight home. I begged them to let me start earlier as I was in a desperate situation. The couple ran an advertising agency in Sydney, so they agreed to give me a temp job in the office until their European trip. They drove me back to the hostel to collect my bags.

While I was out in Australia I contacted Mark and invited him out on holiday. He came out for three weeks and we were able to patch up our relationship. By the time I was ready to leave Sydney I knew I was flying home to my knight in shining armour. When my plane touched down in Heathrow, Mark was there to meet me. Six months later on Friday May 15 1998 we were married. Mum was pleased I had finally settled down, but in her heart perhaps she felt, like many mothers, that the man her daughter was marrying wasn't good enough for her.

Over the years Mark and my mum have had a typical strained mother/son-in-law relationship. She felt that Mark never gave me the support I needed when the children were young and he spent most of his time travelling around the world on business. In the immediate aftermath of the stroke, their relationship was stretched to the limit as they often clashed over my prognosis. They were two different people coming from different sides. For Mark it was all about knowing the facts, no matter how hard they were, and dealing with them for the sake of the family. He was my next of kin and the lynchpin between my family and the medics. But Mum feared that he wasn't telling her the whole story when he said things like,'Still the same. Nothing to report.' She wrote an impassioned letter to the doctors asking if they could meet with her and they agreed. She got the same information but at least she felt happier about being able to ask the doctors directly. Sometimes as I lay in the ICU Mum was upset to see Mark getting on with his family life. What she didn't realise that he was also hurting as deeply as her but had a different method of coping. Eventually, with the intervention of Dave, a man for whom Mark also has great respect, the shared tears and laughter of this traumatic event became the bridge that joined together these two hurt people who loved me most.

Chapter 8
Laughter is the Best Medicine

FOR TEN DAYS AFTER the stroke, while my medical outlook was still bleak, my family had protected well-wishers from the harsh reality of my condition. Initially the only visitors I saw were Mark, Mum and Dave, my dad and his wife, Babs and my in-laws, Ann and Kevin. As the 'ringleader' of my friends Alison had kept in touch with Mark and Mum for regular updates but maintained a respectful distance, not wanting to be seen as interfering or making a nuisance of herself. But as I clung on to life it seemed only right that the friends I had shared so much with in happier times should be allowed back into my world. 'You must go and see her,' Mum urged. Alison made arrangements with Anita to visit.

When I first saw Alison, Anita and Jaqui approach my bed, my eyes said it all: blind panic. They had been fully briefed about my condition, so, I can only imagine the horror going through their minds when they saw me hooked up to the machines keeping me alive. They knew me as Kate the driving force. In my eyes they now saw Kate the frightened victim. The wide grin that I usually wore had gone, replaced by a face that sagged where the muscles could no longer hold it in shape, a mouth that dribbled and eyes that were hollow and scared.

'Hiya, Kate. Guess who bagged the last parking space in the car park? I had to fight off a man in a Range Rover,' Alison proudly announces as she pulls up a chair beside my bed followed by Anita and Jaqui.

I try to smile with my eyes, but fail miserably.

Anita attempts to lift the mood. 'I said to Alison, if this is Kate's way of getting out of boot camp training, she's got another think coming.'

I hear the cheerful banter of my best friend and running buddies and I want to be happy. Theirs is the first laughter I have heard in weeks and I want to join in. But I have an over-riding sense that they are being strong on the surface and underneath they are as scared as I feel, and this worries me. Do they know something I don't? Have they been told my life expectancy? I have no way of asking them.

As my tears started to flow, Alison shot Jaqui and Anita a look as if to say 'Shit, what have we said to upset her?'

'Do you remember that night we got drunk on limoncello?' Alison continues, picking up on something I will respond to. She takes me back to a happier time when our families were together on holidays and having fun. Her talk flows and fills the deathly silence on the ward. Alison is good at talking. It's part of her job. 'Are you going out tonight? Where are you going on holidays?' All stock questions of a hairdresser's trade. Now she's using all her skills to find other inane chatter to fill the void.

'You know you have a reputation as the piss-head of Dore to maintain, so you'd better get well before I steal your crown,' she says reminding me that in their eyes I am still the same person who has shared drunken nights and sober runs together. This makes me feel more positive.

What I did not know at the time was how hard they had found it to actually walk into the ward. Like my mum, they had been standing outside in the waiting room, taking deep breaths and bracing themselves for what lay beyond those swing doors. Alison later likened it to the feeling of an actress going out on stage for the first time. The doors were their curtain, and once they stepped out into the spotlight of the ICU they had to put on a brave face and get on with the show.

As they giggle around my bed I have a feeling that for the first time I am making a connection with them. No words are exchanged but Alison is watching my eyes. She's following my reactions. When I cry she says, 'Kate do you mind if I wipe your face?' before leaning over and mopping up my tears with a paper tissue. When my eyes shut in pain from the cramp, I really believe she is sensing my hurting. We have been reading one another's expressions for so long, surely Alison will say something to the nurses. I am filled with a new hope that my family and the doctors will realise I am alive inside.

When my friends left I watched them walk away, back to their respective homes full of fun and love, and I felt bereft. 'I'll come and see you on Friday before I pick the kids up from school,' Alison says as she departs. I know Alison will not let me down and I hope I cling onto life long enough to see my friends again.

After they had gone, I was left with the nurses and no eye-contact. Once outside the ward, the three of them broke down as they struggled to comfort one another and understand how something so dreadful could happen to one of their own, someone in the prime of her life.

'How can someone so full of life, be so

incapacitated?' Anita asked. 'I can't believe we were having such a laugh at our work-out the morning before it happened and now she may never walk again. It's just not fair.'

After that first visit my friends became regulars, bringing a much-needed injection of life to my gloomy ICU world. I looked forward to their visits. Their bedside manner was always bright and lively, something the doctors and nurses could have taken a lesson from. They never pitied or patronised me, to them I was still Kate – their best mate. They saw beyond my life-support machines and sometimes Alison and Anita would visit, other times Anita brought Jaqui. They would stand at my bedside and I watched as they massaged my feet, which were the only bits of me that didn't have some kind of tube or wire attached. They were able to carry out the caring and compassionate acts when the nursing staff were just too busy to notice. Sometimes Alison came alone and sat by my bedside and read chapters from the current book from our book group.

She would lift my spirits with stories from her hectic life at the salon and her chaotic nights on the town with her hairdressing friends.

'It's snowing outside,' she announced one afternoon in late February. 'Shall we take your bed outside and use it like a sledge?' I was reminded of one playful morning the previous winter when Alison and I had taken the children to school to be told they could go home. It had been snowing heavily overnight and any parents who were worried about getting their children home safely were allowed to take them out of class early. If we had been responsible mums we would have taken advantage of the school's concern and done just that. But the wintry downfall brought out the big kids in us and we left the children in school and rushed home, dug out Harvey's sledge from the toy cupboard, put on our ski clothes, packed a flask of milky coffee and some of my home-made flapjacks and headed for a farmer's field. There was no one about, which is just as well as for three hours we skidded back to our childhood, careering down the snowy hill on a wooden toboggan. If anyone had seen us they'd probably have thought we were a couple of care in the community cases. We laughed ourselves silly as we created a 'sledge sandwich' with me drawing the short straw and going on the bottom to steer with Alison sitting on top of me.

My eyes sparkle at this talk of our snowy adventure and I want to remind her how I still haven't forgiven her for jumping off half-way down and leaving me to ride straight into a bush.

I hope there will be more outdoor adventures in future. Again Alison is watching my expression, I am convinced she is thinking the same: that we will be back to our old tricks one day. Outside the hospital, my friends spent many long hours searching for answers to my condition. 'I'm sure that Kate understands what we are saying. The way she reacts to our silly stories can't be a coincidence,' Alison suggested.

They swotted up on other cases of locked-in syndrome and young stroke patients, they read books written by other extreme cases and they talked to my family about little signs they thought they had detected and discussed ways they could help.

Chapter 9
Two Blinks for Yes, One for No

THREE WEEKS AFTER THE stroke came the breakthrough I had been waiting for.

'Kate can you understand what I'm saying? Blink twice if you can?' Mark asked. I could not believe it, I was being asked a question and given the opportunity to reply. I blinked, slowly and deliberately. One. Two. When I opened my eyes the second time Mark was looking at me with the widest, daftest grin on his face I've ever seen. 'Do it again,' he encouraged me. I did.

'Thank fuck for that,' I thought to myself as he called to the efficient older nurse who was busy filling out a chart on the bed opposite. I had been so frustrated by the lack of communication it felt as though someone had put a microphone up to my mouth for the world to hear, I could 'talk'.

'Kate, can you understand me?' the nurse says, slowly and considerately. Again I blink twice and I wish I had the means to say, 'And I'm not stupid, so you don't have to speak like I'm an imbecile.'

'Are you comfortable?' the nurse asks. 'Blink once for no and twice for yes. I blink once. I am not comfortable. Are you in pain? One blink for no. Not at the moment, anyway. 'Are you hot?' Yes. I blink twice and she switches on a fan beside my bed. I cry with relief. I want to reach out and hug Mark for being my mouthpiece.

I now knew that all my worst nightmares, about being treated as a vegetable for the rest of my life, or having my life support switched off, were not going to come true.

While I had never really given up hope, from that moment my natural optimism and fighting spirit could reassert themselves and I started to have real hope that I would get better.

It transpired that Mark had been paying more attention to my reactions than I gave him credit for. When I was watching the television at the bottom of my bed he noticed how I seemed to avert my eyes when a programme I hated came on. When he talked to me about his day at work and the people who were getting him down, he saw I was rolling my eyes in sympathy. When he talked about the children I would cry. This was no coincidence. At home he had talked to Alison and she had shared her own feelings that I was understanding everything that was going on.

When Mark and I were left alone again, he explained what had happened. 'Kate you've had a stroke,' were his only words. This made no sense to me. In my mind strokes were something that only happened to old people and people who had them were left paralysed down one side of the body. Why was I completely paralysed? Strangely, for someone who is normally so inquisitive, I didn't want to know any more detail and Mark did not elaborate.

As a result of this advancement in communication a card was placed by the side of my bed.

2 blinks = yes
1 blink = no

One afternoon Alison arrived for her usual visit accompanied by a very official-looking man and woman, in suits. I started to panic and Alison had to calm me down. Was I being asked to sign my will? Did they know I was about to die? Morbid thoughts were racing through my mind, which weren't so irrational considering that all the medical staff and my family were protecting me from my poor prognosis. Alison explained that Mark had instructed a company of Sheffield solicitors to arrange a lasting power of attorney. Mark could not be there to influence the process and had asked Alison to act as the witness. For Mark it was another of those steps in keeping life on track. We had a joint critical illness insurance policy that required both our signatures to make a claim. We also had a joint bank account and with the other party incapable of nodding her head, let alone signing her name, he was thinking ahead and getting our finances in order. By appointing him as my 'Attorney' while I was incapable of doing something as simple as writing a cheque or signing a letter, he would be able to look after our finances and home. I remembered that Mark had told me about it on a previous visit, but I didn't expect it to come as such a blow. The whole time I was in the ICU I had the impression that I was waiting on Death Row. I believed I was going to die, I just didn't know when or how, and I felt those around me knew it too.

Alison introduced me to the solicitors and they held a sheet of paper in front of my eyes to read. They already had a certificate signed by the consultant neurologist that confirmed I was suffering from locked-in syndrome and was unable to speak. He said he was 'certain that I had the capacity to make decisions for myself provided communication was via eye movement and blinking and that although I could not sign a Lasting Power of Attorney, I was capable of authorising a third party. In this case Alison was the third party. She asked me a series of questions, which she read to me from the official document, and I had to blink if I agreed. Then she signed for me, and again I had to blink my consent.

When the official deed was done the suits walked out, leaving Alison to pick up the pieces.

'It's only a formality. There's no need to worry, it's just one of those legal things that Mark needs to make sure he can sign things on your behalf and look after your finances,' she reassured me. I wasn't convinced. In my mind the message was loud and clear, if you need to hand over control of your financial affairs you're on your way out. No one had told me so, but the voices in my head were telling me, 'Goodnight. That's your lot.' Alison stayed with me longer than usual, worried about leaving me in such a state. When the time came for her to finally say goodnight, I was crying deeper and longer than I had ever before. As she walked out I really felt that she was saying her last goodbye. I thought back to the conversation Mark and I had had when we had been talking about the need for us to finalise our wills in case anything should happen to us, and he had said he would want to be 'finished off' from his misery if something happened to him and he was left brain-dead. I was now scared that Mark had made that decision on my behalf.

I lost the will to live. I really, really wished Mark would come and put that pillow over my head. For days I sank into a real depression, I couldn't be bothered talking to my visitors and felt they were all there to say their last goodbyes.

It was Alison who brought me out of my black mood with one of her usual cheerful and charitable visits. I had been suffering from a particularly long and painful cramp attack when Alison walked in. Immediately I was so relieved to see her, in the hope she would help me. Seeing my sad eyes, she asked 'Are you in pain?' Two blinks for yes. A primary school-level lesson in biology followed as she pointed to each part of my body watching for the all-important two blinks. Once we had located the area of discomfort, my legs, she asked, 'Is it an ache?' Two blinks. 'Is it cramp?' Off she went to ask a nurse to remove my leg braces so that she could spend the rest of the visiting session massaging my aching limbs. My friends soon began to realise that cramp was one of the things that was dragging me down. Some afternoons I would be in so much pain, I'd cry with relief when I saw them walk in. They soon understood that cramp was the likely cause of my tears and gently moved my legs to ease the pain. Other methods of diagnosis involved 'Do you need medication?' Two blinks. 'Do you need something now?' One blink for no. 'Do you need something soon?' Two blinks. At these times Alison would go off and ask if I could be given a dose of painkillers. Another time it was just that my hot, sweaty leg braces were causing an unbearable itching sensation that I was powerless to scratch. Again Alison would pinpoint the problem with a series of yes/no questions and get on with scratching my itch. Heaven.

Encouraged by this basic method of communication, my friends put their heads together and devised a pain chart. The idea had come from a conversation Anita and Alison had been having with a group of mums.

One of our friends, who taught autistic children, suggested that a technique they used at her school might work for me too. Anita drew a crude line drawing of figure with the questions: Need something now? Need something soon? Pain? Ache? Sore? Front, back, side, top? Discomfort? Itch? Massage? Medication?

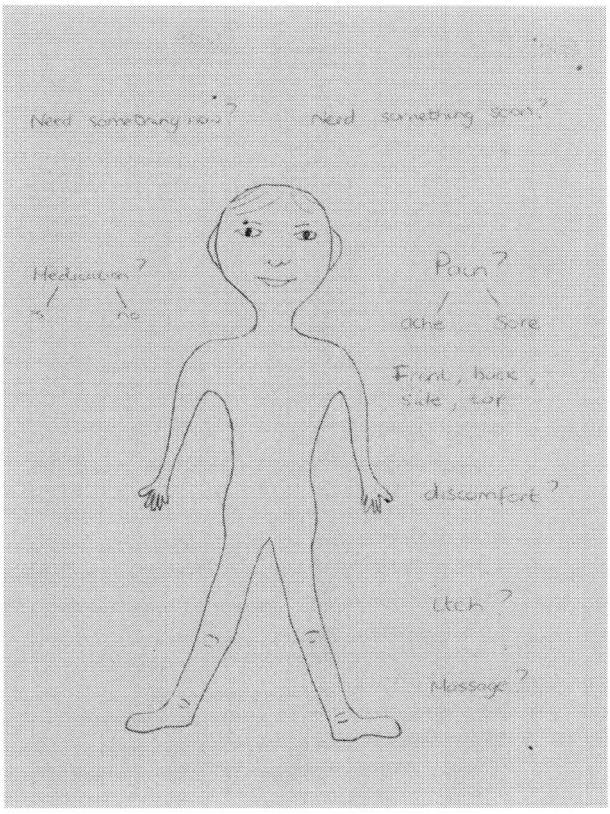

Yes? No? The little person drawn in red ink with big bulging red eyes looked more like an alien than a human. I guess art isn't Anita's strong point, but it made me smile and did the trick. The chart became the mantra for all my visitors who were effectively able to become the voice of need.

I had waited for more than three weeks, but now I

was able to express the things that were getting me down as long as there was someone willing to spell out the chart. Alison, Anita and Jaqui would take the time to sit with me and work their way through the various pain combinations until they saw the look in my eyes that said, 'Thank you.'

From this the girls advanced to a letter board containing every letter of the alphabet. They had read many books and articles on the subject of strokes and locked-in syndrome and it seemed that many patients were able to improve their communication using such a device. During their visits, Alison, Anita and Jaqui came armed with their alphabet and we would spend the next hour or so trying to spell out words. It was a slow and painstaking means of communication. Every letter had to be pronounced clearly and they would have to wait for a reaction. A simple three or four-letter word took at least 20 minutes to spell out. One of the first messages I blinked was 'CAN'T SLEEP'. 'You can't sleep?' Jaqui queried. I blinked twice. 'At night?' she ventured. Again I blinked twice. 'You're saying you can't sleep at night.' Again I blinked twice. At last someone could understand me. That night I was given a dose of crushed sleeping pills and for the first time ever I slept right through the night from 11 p.m. to 6 a.m.

I now understand how sleep deprivation can be used as a means of torture. After my first proper sleep, my whole outlook on life brightened. Having this channel to convey my needs was a great relief and gave me hope that I might be included in my treatment. If my family and the nurses knew my mind was working, there was no way they would switch off the machines and leave me to die without asking me first.

I very quickly learnt that the communication board was

only as effective as the person on the other end. If I had no one to read the alphabet, I had no voice. I also discovered that some of my family and friends and even the nurses were more patient than others when it came to struggling to understand my needs. The worst offender was my mum who would pick up the chart and read out the letters, but her eyes would wander off to other parts of the ward while I was blinking for all I was worth.

'Look at me or put it down,' I wanted to shout at her as my energy drained. It took an enormous amount of effort to spell out a short word when Mum drifted off, I would just close my eyes and sulk. That's when I realised where I inherited my impatience from.

Alison was pretty bad too, but at least she tried to keep focussed on the job in hand. A B C D E ... and so she would make her way through the alphabet until I blinked twice on the letter O. She misread this as a letter P. Then we walked through the letters again adding a U and a T. 'PUT?' You want me to put something ...?' she quizzed. 'No I want to go OUT,' I was trying to tell her. 'I want to OUTSIDE.' 'You want me to put something ...' It was useless I couldn't get through. I stared hard at the fire door opposite my bed that led out into a courtyard. I sensed life beyond the tempered glass. I was desperate to go outside and feel the fresh air on my face. It was the end of February and the temperature outside was close to freezing, but I yearned to escape from the stifling, stagnant atmosphere of the ICU.

Alison has been friends with me long enough to know that when I wanted something badly, I stared. We have this bond where sometimes words are unnecessary, which is lucky as we were getting nowhere fast with our word board. So I fixed my eyes on the door. This led to a game of ICU charades. Alison leapt around the ward touching things and asking 'Am I warm?' I would blink if she was right. She touched the fan beside my bed. I blinked once for no and stared at the fire door. She pointed to my feet indicating a massage. No, I blinked, and stared at the door. She pointed to the TV suggesting I might want to switch the channel from an afternoon chat show to a cookery programme. Again I blinked no and stared at the door. Finally the penny dropped and she stood by the door. Yes, I blinked. 'You want to go outside?' she asked. Yes, I blinked. 'At last,' I thought. Alison once again became my mouthpiece and went off in search of a nurse. It wasn't an easy task but one that Alison was determined to make happen as she understood that something as simple as the sensation of the icy wind on my cheeks would be more therapeutic to me than any amount of super-strength painkillers.

My physiotherapists had already started to hoist me in and out of a support chair during my therapy sessions. Now a major removal exercise began as the hoist was wheeled to my bed and I was heaved like a lifeless soul into a sturdy, padded chair on wheels, like those they use in old people's homes. Slumped in the chair, with pillows propping up my body, breathing/feeding tube combo on wheels beside me I was moved outside. All my tubes and pipes were adjusted and a nurse accompanied us to monitor the machines. The courtyard wasn't the most picturesque place in the world. The views over a low wall into a car park didn't compare with the view over the valleys of Baslow and Hathersage from the top of the Peaks. But it was a window on a world where life was carrying on as normal, people were going about their everyday business, and when I had spent a month in an environment of death and sadness this was an enormous boost to my morale. Once I had a taste of life on the outside, I wanted more. I was happy to sit outside for two or three hours at a time. I was snuggled up warm beneath my blankets, it was my poor visitors who were shivering in the cold. But we would always try and see the funny and ridiculous side of life. I remember on one occasion one of the nurses without thinking said, 'shout me if you need me'. Mark laughed out loud and I tried to force a smile.

Of all my visitors only Jaqui seemed to have the diligence to really get to grips with the letter board and even in her capable hands, I found the whole process exhausting. I mastered several key words like OUT, HOT and SLEEP to convey my discomfort and TEA to get across that I was desperate for a cuppa even though I was still not allowed to drink.

This laborious letter chart was short-lived as the nurses advised my friends it was not suitable system as they used a different colour-coded chart for patients learning to communicate and thought that this might confuse me later in my rehabilitation. So the alphabet was withdrawn. In some ways I was relieved as it was more hassle than it was worth and I found my eyes became a more reliable way of getting the message across.

I started looking forward to my friends' visits, they were always fun and took my mind off my dire situation. Alison often sat by my bed and read stories to me from the daily newspaper or she would bring along the book she was reading and recite extracts. One day she read me Warren Beatty's autobiography but stopped at the more salacious bits.

'I think the man in the next bed is getting a bit too excited,' she whispered.

As soon as the doctors realised my mind was unaffected and I could respond to questions with blinks they started to involve me in my treatment. One morning I was asked if I was willing for them to perform a tracheotomy. Basically they wanted to slit my throat and insert a tube which would help me breathe. For me it was a no-brainer as it would mean I'd finally be rid of the tube that was filling my mouth and causing me constant discomfort. I blinked twice for yes. My mum, however, had been dead against the operation and resisted it on my behalf until this point. She believed that, once in, it would never be taken out. She had a friend who had died with a 'trachi' as it's commonly known. From her experience she believed that it was the beginning of the end and the trachi would bring complications like an increased risk of infection and even pneumonia, the big killer of locked-in patients, so she understandably dug in her heels. I, on the other hand, believed the doctors when they said it was only a temporary measure until I was able to breathe for myself. It didn't cross my mind that this might be a permanent measure – I just wanted the tubes out of my mouth.

The doctors warned that the operation carried a high risk of damaging my vocal chords. I could be left with a hoarse voice, or no voice at all. Even this didn't worry me. At the time I did not know they had predicted I would never walk or talk again, as they were protecting me from my own prognosis. But in my head I had played over this killer question in the quiz show of life. Faced with the choice, would you rather walk or talk? I always chose walk. For me running and activity were more important than speech. Don't get me wrong, the old Kate could talk for Yorkshire but I truly believed that there were many other ways to communicate – there was only one way to run. So, the following day I was taken down to the operating theatre and the operation was performed under anaesthetic. I kept the trachi in for nine weeks.

A week later I was taken back to the operating theatre, this time I was to have a PEG fitted. A PEG, in doc-speak, is a 'percutaneous endoscopic gastrostomy', which to me sounded like a dish Heston Blumenthal might cook. A PEG was actually a good description of what was inserted into the left-hand side of my body. It was a hollow plastic peg and looked like something you would buy in a camping shop. It's a common procedure for stroke patients whose swallowing is impaired.

I could now be fed directly through the tube into my stomach at four-hourly intervals, rather than the tube up my nose. It was one less tube to irritate me and it would also cut the risk of developing pneumonia, which I had learned was the main killer for sufferers of severe strokes like mine.

Chapter 10
Eighteen Again

EACH TIME MY FRIENDS Alison, Anita and Jaqui came to see me they would struggle with conversation. What could they talk about? For them the idea of telling me about all the routine things they had been doing and the great runs they had been on seemed too cruel when I was completely paralysed and going nowhere.

So conversation always reverted to my children. Keen not to say thoughtless things that might upset me, my friends would come in with a script in their head of safe, if one-sided, subjects for conversation and top of that list was the children. They'd chat about the things India, Harvey and Woody had been up to, daft, harmless little things that only a mother would notice. And this was the most painful conversation of all. I had to lie there and listen to how they were getting on with their lives – without me. I hated it. It upset me to know that I had been their main carer all their lives and now I could do nothing for them. I could not hug them, or talk to them, or even reach out to touch them. Hearing about them just made me feel bereft and hollow. All I wanted to know was that they were OK and that they were still maintaining some kind of routine by going to their regular activities: football for Harvey, Beavers and piano lessons for Woody and Girl Guides for India. It was the only way I could deal with a situation that was killing me inside. My eyes would glaze over and I drifted away to a time when I was a non-mother.

In my head I was eighteen again. I was leaving home and heading for America to be a nanny. It was December 1988 and I found myself with a year to fill. I had exceeded my teachers' and parents' expectations by passing my A levels with decent grades. Two Bs and a D in economics, business and social studies meant I had made the grade for university. There was just one problem – as everyone expected me to fail big time I had not applied to any. With my grades I was offered a place on the business studies course at Sheffield Polytechnic the following September, so I had a year to fill with boring office temping jobs.

One day I was reading *The Lady* when I spotted an advert for an au pair agency in London. Sensing an opportunity for adventure, I convinced Dave to take me to London for an interview. We were driving back home to Macclesfield when the agency called to say they had a job for me … in Washington, Virginia.

But this trip almost ended in disaster before it had begun. I booked my ticket on Pan Am Flight 103 from Heathrow to New York's JFK Airport on Wednesday December 21. But as the leaving date drew closer I realised I wanted to spend Christmas with my family and called the airline to postpone my flight until the new year. It turned out to be a lucky escape as all 243 passengers and sixteen flight staff were killed when a bomb exploded on the Boeing 747 as it flew over a Scottish town in what would forever be known as the Lockerbie Disaster.

On January 4 I said a tearful goodbye to Mum, Dad and Dave at the departure gate at Heathrow, as I jetted off for a new life in a new country living with a family I had never met. In a sense I was running away. I had been dumped by my first serious boyfriend, Mark I, and my heart was still in pieces. We had been together for three years and before he came on the scene I had no interest in boys. I had two brothers and all boys were annoying and definitely something to be avoided. America was my chance to forget and face up to a new challenge with new people. My dad told me I would hate it and be back on the next flight. Mum cried, partly because she felt she was losing her elder daughter, but also perhaps because she was jealous that I had the guts to seize opportunities as they came. When she was my age she was married and already a mother to my brother Paul. She was also worried about my safety. It was less than two weeks after the Lockerbie bombing I had so narrowly missed, there were armed police at the airport security gates and Britain was on its first high terror alert. As I left she handed me a letter, which I tucked away in my bra. It read 'Kate, we love you very much and will miss you. Don't ever feel you are stuck. If you need money or want to come home just call us. We'll always be there for you. Lots of love, Mum and Dave.'

After a month I did call them – to invite them out on holiday. My employers lived on a huge ranch in the Virginia countryside where they bred and rode racehorses. He was a lawyer who loved the English and shooting turkeys. She was a rich housewife who spent her days being pampered and playing tennis with her coach. They had a four-year-old son and an eighteen-month-old daughter, and it was my responsibility to look after them by day. I could never understand why they needed me there when their mother didn't work. I vowed to myself that when I had children, as I hoped I would one day when I met Mr Right, I would always be there for them.

During the six months I lived in Virginia I was lonely. I lived in a large attic room in the house and had everything I could need, except companionship. The ranch was five miles away from the nearest house and it was hard to make friends. Sometimes I went alone to the bars of Middleberg, an extremely Anglophile town where the locals would come and befriend me on hearing my accent.

One couple, Sam and Gladys, took me under their wing. They were old-school southerners. Sam drank bourbon for breakfast and went hunting for worms for fishing at dawn. Gladys was homely and baked me a cake for my birthday. They were like my surrogate parents and showed their southern hospitality when Mum and Dave came to visit me. While in America I also found love, or that's what I thought at the time, with Will. I met him when he visited the ranch to ride; he was a member of the Olympic equestrian team in Boston and ten years older than me. I thought he was the one and that we would be together for ever. I was wrong. When I returned to England we lost touch and I threw myself into college life.

On these occasions when my mind switched back to happier times, when I had no one dependent on me, it was my only means of coping with the separation anxiety. At first my friends could not understand why I seemed to be switching off every time they mentioned India, Harvey or Woody. They could not grasp why I seemed to be losing interest and drifting off during the carefully scripted conversations.

For days my behaviour was the subject of great debates among my friends until they finally twigged that it was the talk of my children that seemed to be the trigger. For them it was impossible to imagine why I would not want to know what my children were doing.

They had their fully functioning families and there could be no greater social taboo than a mother who did not put her children first in her thoughts and actions. Jaqui, as ever the one to think 'outside the box', suggested that maybe I did not want to hear so much detail about my children's lives. 'Maybe Kate cannot cope knowing she is unable to be a mother to her children. We can't know how she is feeling and should not relate our normal social standards and judgement to Kate's situation,' Jaqui suggested to Alison and Anita one evening after they had left the ward. Slowly the idea began to sink in that we have a finite capacity to care and that capacity is determined by how well we are able to function. In my case all I could do was manage the day-to-day traumas of surviving, I wasn't able to worry about anyone else, even my own children. It was not that I did not care, I was simply unable to care, and once my friends came to their own reasoned understanding of that, our one-way conversations became less awkward.

Chapter 11
Mummy's Only Crying Because She's Happy to See You

MY SPIRIT WAS LIFTED by a visit from my daughter India. Throughout his daily routine from work to hospital and home, the biggest issue eating away at Mark was whether he should bring our children in to see me. In the weeks that followed my stroke, the children had been struggling with an upset home routine where they were being cared for by an emotionally exhausted dad.

The stress was beginning to show on all my immediate family. India was suffering from sickness and skin problems brought on by anxiety and Woody and Harvey were rebelling against their nana and grandma who were sharing the duty of surrogate mum. Woody would constantly throw tantrums and Mark's mother found him difficult to control. Harvey said hurtful things to his grandparents, for example when he saw my mum putting her slippers on the stairs he told her in no uncertain terms to 'take them away, they don't belong there'. He had noticed that strange slippers on the stairs meant another night without his mum.

I was out of the coma and didn't look quite as dead as I had but I was still in a shocking state. Mark guessed I would like to see them but was concerned that the sight of their mum looking not much better than Frankenstein's monster might have a traumatic effect on them. Mark worked for a company producing wound-care dressings, so he was used to dealing with doctors and medical professionals. Over a period of two weeks he asked each of the sixteen consultants in the ICU for advice on whether bringing three young children in to see their mother was a good idea. And their advice was all pretty much the same – useless. When it came to a personal issue there was no guidebook to follow. Afraid of putting themselves in a potentially liable situation, they all trotted out the same tried and tested answer that there were no guidelines and only Mark could know how his children would react. This wasn't enough for the father who wanted to do the right thing by his fragile family and he pressed each one with the words, 'Put yourself in my shoes, my friend, what would you do?' His persistent words must have struck a chord with the professionals, many were men in their forties and I can only imagine they were thinking, there but for the grace of God. One by one they all admitted that if they were in Mark's shoes they would allow their children to visit.

That was all he needed. The following day mummy's girl India, the 'mother of my tribe', made an appearance on the ward. India has always been older and wiser than her years and if truth were told she was more of a support for her dad than she realised. When she walked into the ward for the first time, I cried. My little Indi was as strong as an ox; inside she was hurting, but she sat at the side of my bed for forty-five minutes, gently stroking my arm, and proceeded to tell me what she had done at school that day, just as if I was 'regular mum' standing in the kitchen cooking tea. After a while the heat and stifling, stagnant airlessness took its toll and India started to feel unwell. Mark's mum took her outside and she was sick with the shock.

A week later Harvey visited with Mark and his mum. This trip was even more difficult as Harvey is your typical football- and rugby-playing ten-year-old boy. On the outside he looks and acts tough, a bundle of boyish energy always arguing with his younger brother. But inside he's surprisingly sensitive. After India's successful visit, Mark asked Harvey if he wanted to see me and the answer was a straightforward, 'No, I'm not ready.' This hurt Mark but he didn't want to force the issue, it was up to Harvey to make a decision in his own time. When he was ready he asked Mark one afternoon on the car ride home from school, 'Can I go and see Mum tomorrow?'

On the journey to the hospital Harvey asked about India's visit.

'Dad, if I'm struggling can I ask for a time out? I don't want to upset Mum.' Here was a 10-year-old boy wanting to protect his protector from his own vulnerability. Harvey didn't ask for time out. He sat beside the bed and talked to me and stroked my hand while I cried. When visiting time was over he left. In the car on the way back home he cried in silence. When he got home he went to bed and cried. But his tears were like no others Mark had seen. He made no noise, but the tears flowed. When he got up for school the next morning, he was still tearful and emotional. Mark became worried that he had caused irreparable emotional damage by exposing him to the death and illness of the ICU. When Harvey got home from school that afternoon, he had stopped crying and he was back to his usual self, much to Mark's relief. He couldn't talk about it but from that moment on; he had come to terms with the situation and was able to accept my illness.

Woody was the most difficult to deal with. The baby

of the family, he was only six and missing his mum's hugs and kisses. His older brother and sister had already told him about their visits, so who knows what was going through his young mind. 'Will Mummy know me?' he asked Mark on the journey to the hospital. Mark replied, 'Yes, but she might cry because she is happy to see you.' When Woody's face appeared at the side of my bed, the tears started rolling down my face. I wanted so much to give him a hug and all I could do to show him how much I loved him was cry. The bloody health and safety brigade wouldn't even let the kids sit on the edge of my bed so I could feel their touch. It was all wrong. My little Woody stood beside me and stroked my arm. On the way home, Woody cried too.

The visits had been a tearful time for all the family. But it was one more positive mental step on my road to recovery. As the weeks passed, Mark and the kids took it in turns to sit and mop my brow with cotton wool and Simple toner. I loved the contact and in time visits became more relaxed.

Chapter 12
Time for Tea

WITH MY FEEDING PEG fitted the 'Nil by Mouth' sign remained over my bed. I got attached to a feeding bag at four-hourly intervals for my nutrition. It was better than a tube up the nose, but it was nowhere near as comforting as a cup of Earl Grey tea.

'I bet you fancy a cup of tea,' the Stoke nurse said to me one afternoon as she busied herself tending my life-preserving machines. She was not wrong and I blinked twice for yes. For days I had been staring at the box of Earl Grey tea bags that Mark had brought in for me knowing it was one of the few things that might bring a fraction of normality to my life.

Unfortunately it wasn't simply a case of switching on the kettle and popping a tea bag into a cup. What followed was a major task to determine if I could actually drink tea without it killing me. One of the main concerns for stroke patients is a condition called silent aspiration, which can be deadly. In simple terms it is food and drink going down the wrong way. A normal person would just cough the obstruction back up, but as I had no coughing or choking reflex there was no way of telling if tea was going down the wrong pipe. And if this did happen it could lead to a chest infection or pneumonia, which could be the end of me.

Was it worth risking my life for? I thought so, but the medical staff had to be careful. The Stoke nurse spoke to a senior nurse, who spoke to a doctor and they agreed that first of all they would give me a food dye to make sure the liquids were going down the right pipe and into my stomach and not my lungs. One of the nurses dripped five drops of food dye onto my tongue and let it trickle down my throat. Then they hoovered my lungs to make sure the dye hadn't taken a wrong turn. This was a pretty foul experience. It began with a nurse taking the cap off the end of my trachi pipe and inserting their 'hoover'. I could feel the ferocity of the machine as it sucked everything up from inside my lungs while all the time the machine made disgusting gurgling sounds like a giant coffee percolator. Once they were satisfied that the mucous they had hoovered from my lungs was clear, they knew the dye was going down my gullet and not my windpipe, and the Stoke nurse brought me a cup of tea in a beaker.

I had hoped for Earl Grey with sugar and milk, what I actually got was Yorkshire tea with milk and no sugar, but I couldn't complain. It was progress. At first I could not actually taste the tea, I could just feel the sensation of the heat as the liquid passed over my tongue, a few drops at a time. The nurse tipped the beaker into my mouth allowing gravity to drag it down into my throat as my mouth and oesophagus muscles were inactive. After every four or five mouthfuls the Stoke nurse stopped and got the hoover out and suck to ensure my lungs were empty. Then after five rounds of drops and suction the nurses would abandon the tea drinking and get on with their other work. I was always gutted when they stopped. It may have seemed like a long and drawn-out process for my twice daily cup of tea, but for me it was worth all the discomfort just to have that feeling of normality. It gave me hope that one day I would be able to drink without the hoover.

Chapter 13
A Lie a Day Keeps ICU Away

TIME DRAGGED IN THE ICU. I had defied the odds against survival and made significant, albeit minor, advances in communication. Once I was off the critical list, the next stage would be a lengthy rehabilitation to accept and learn to live with my severe disabilities.

Osborn 4, the rehabilitation ward, was in a separate building on the hospital site. As none of the doctors believed I would walk or talk again it was more a case of moving on to free up a bed. However in my mind the move to a different ward was a huge psychological step forward. It meant that I was able to escape from the depressing environment of death row. With a new ward would come new staff. I firmly believed there were certain members of staff on the ICU ward who only pretended to 'care' for me when my visitors were around and wanted me dead. Getting accepted on to the Osborn 4 unit had been a battle in itself. Being a rehab ward it only took patients who were showing signs of reactions to stimuli and, by definition, receptive to rehabilitation therapy. With almost no signs of movement, the doctors wanted to move me onto the specialist stroke ward until my family dug their heels in. They believed that on a specialist rehabilitation ward my speech and mobility would be assessed and I'd get the intensive therapy I needed to help me relearn all the functions I had lost. On the stroke ward I might miss out on a lot of this therapy.

To determine whether I was ready to make the move, doctors had a test which they carried out to check if the brain was functioning and able to sense smell. That way they could assess if new paths were developing inside my brain. At this point I couldn't actually smell a thing, but I knew the routine as I had watched several patients being tested over the course of the weeks. The doctor waved an alcohol wipe in front of my nose and right on cue I flinched, just the slightest twitch to show I was reacting to the sharp smell. Next he waved a cloth, which had been dipped in vinegar, below my nostrils and I repeated the movement closing my eyes tightly to indicate I was sensitive to the acrid smell. Truth was I couldn't smell a thing but I had watched out of the corner of my eye as he took the wipe out of the box labelled 'alcohol wipes' and dipped the other cloth in a vinegar bottle. If any of the doctors had taken the time to get to know me while I was on their ward they would have realised that I might have been 'locked-in' but I wasn't stupid and my brain was working overtime.

There was just one problem, once I had passed the necessary test I still had to wait. There was a lack of beds on Osborn 4 as many of the patients were there long-term with spinal and brain injuries and beds were at a premium.

Four times I had my hopes raised only to find there were no beds available and I would have to stay in the ICU. Then late one Friday evening after Mark had left and Anita was my last visitor of the night, I had the news I was waiting for. I could go. It was a delicate operation. The machines that were breathing and feeding me had to move too. The ambulance was booked and I would be moving in four hours. It seemed like an odd time to be shifting, but I didn't care, I was just happy to leave. I couldn't move the muscles in my face to smile, but inside I was delighted. Anita could see the joy in my eyes and broke out in a Cheshire-cat grin big enough for both of us. She called Mark from her mobile to break the good news, which must have been as much of a surprise to him as it was to me as when he left an hour earlier there was no indication that I would be moving that night.

I didn't care that it was late; it wasn't as if I had any more pressing engagements. I was leaving death row. As the ICU staff and porters gathered my belongings one of the nurses came up to say goodbye.

'Best of luck, you'll not see me again,' she said. And then came out with words that were to leave a lasting impression on me. 'I used to work on Osborn 4 and I'm warning you now, they will push you hard in rehab so be prepared to work hard.'

Game on. I was ready for a challenge.

Chapter 14
Welcome to Osborn 4

I ARRIVED ON THE new ward like a stranger in the night with an entourage of porters and nurses.

Osborn 4 was based in the spinal wing of the hospital and was one of the main rehabilitation wards for patients who had suffered major head injuries. Named after our former Sheffield Hallam MP Sir John Holbrook Osborn, the ward was divided, with a nursing station in the centre. Leading off it were three bays, each with four beds, and two private rooms to which everyone aspired. As time passed I understood that the further away from the nurses' station your bed was, the better your chances of going home.

I was wheeled into the high-dependency unit, a two-bed ward right under the noses of the medical staff. I understood this as code for being pretty poorly. The woman lying in the bed opposite me was seriously ill. I never found out what was wrong with her but she looked as if she had suffered a car accident or some other major trauma. She was about forty-five, unable to speak, and wore a helmet which looked as if she had a serious head injury. When it came to meal times she had to be spoon-fed like a baby but at least, for all her problems, she could eat and drink, which was more than I could. As soon as I'd arrived disaster had struck and my Earl Grey tea was withdrawn because it was trickling into my lungs and slowly killing me.

Don't get me wrong, Osborn 4 was no five-star hotel but I hoped it would become my own clinical equivalent of a health spa. In reality it was to become more like a prison cell, with the occasional time out for good behaviour. For the time being I was just glad to be away from the oppressive atmosphere and overriding gloominess of the ICU.

If my rehabilitation was to be a success, it was hugely important to set myself goals. The journey ahead was long and as my friend Jaqui always used to say, 'You can't eat an elephant whole, you have to take bite-sized chunks.' For me those early goals sounded small but were in fact huge: sitting up; moving my hand in order to relieve an itch, call for help and hold a pen; standing upright; breathing without a tube and drinking liquids again. Longer term in my mind I wanted to walk and talk; eat proper food; go home to live; be a mum again and go for a run.

The move on to Osborn 4 had been a goal ticked off my list. I had been told that I was going to be moved to a halfway ward, to acclimatise patients who were fresh out of intensive care before moving on to rehab. As there were no empty beds we cut out the middle move.

When the shifts changed that first night on Osborn 4 I encountered my first night terror – Lorna. She was one of the older nurses, a mountain of a woman who terrified me. 'Bloody hell, what have I moved to?' I thought to myself that night as Lorna waddled around the ward with her menacing mannerisms. It was two months before she even looked me in the eye. In her presence I always felt like it was my fault I had ended up in the state I was in. The first few weeks on the new ward were a case of me being weaned off the one-to-one care of the ICU and slowly eased into a programme of physiotherapy. Nothing very much had changed in my physical well-being. I was still breathing with a ventilator, being fed through a PEG and drained through a catheter. I could do nothing for myself. But there had been a flicker of movement in my right thumb while I was in the ICU. This had been spotted by my physiotherapist while he was puzzling over what to do with me during our regular sessions. 'That's a good sign,' he enthused in his thick New Zealand accent. It had only happened once and therefore was too slight to be of any real significance, but it was an indication that new pathways might be opening up and sending messages from my brain to my muscles. However my rehab team were of the opinion that any movement that did come back would be incidental not functional. So I might be able to move a thumb, but I could not hold a pen or wipe my arse.

During that time the medical staff also came to the conclusion that I was crying because I was grieving for the life I had lost. In fact, like a baby, I had learned that crying brought you attention and crying was the only method of communication I had control over. Consequently, like an infant, if I felt that warm, unpleasant sensation of a full nappy I'd cry and hope the nurses would pick up on the smell and come and change me. At other times, if I was too hot and needed the fan to cool me down, I would cry. When I was uncomfortable from lying in the same position for hours on end and needed to be turned to relieve the pressure on my sore joints, I cried. This should have been done every four hours, but sometimes the nurses forgot and it would feel like a lifetime lying there, unable to move in order to ease the pressure. That was one of the most cruel things about being locked in, I could feel pain, even though my body was completely paralysed and powerless to ease it.

My crying reminded me of a time when Woody was only a few months old and Alison had thrown a pampering pyjama party for me and the girls. My mum had agreed to babysit for India and Harvey and I had taken Woody along with me. It was the first time I had been out since having him and after a couple of glasses of wine I was feeling a little the worse for wear. I went upstairs to the bathroom to wash the mud pack off my face, having put a sleeping Woody down on Alison's spare bed en route. When I had finished in the bathroom I returned downstairs to my friends and carried on drinking and laughing. No one noticed Woody was missing until we heard him crying in the bedroom. When I ran up I saw how dangerously close to the edge of the bed he was.

During my time on Osborn 4 I made some great friends among the nursing staff, who were heartbroken that something so drastic should have happened to someone as young and fit as me. For some, who were mothers too, I couldn't help but think that my predicament made them realise just how cruel the lottery of life could be.

It seemed that one of the qualifications for nursing on Osborn 4 was having the name Sara. There were three of them. Sara 'Dark Hair' was the sister who very early on realised that I was going to be a rule-breaker and as a result treated me more like an equal than a patient. Then there was Sara 'Bob', a rather stern woman who had been nursing for two decades and was efficient, but cold and clinical. When I first arrived on the ward I craved compassion and warmth from the nurses and all I got from her was rules and regulations.

As my condition improved and I became less needy I responded to her matter-of-fact nature. Her best friend was a stocky woman also called Sara. I called her 'Sara Short'; she was the opposite of 'Bob' and would react when I cried. Regardless of whether I was really sad or just seeking attention, she always responded. She was the one I trusted most to change my nappies and sort out my pads when my 'monthlies' came around. At night time there was 'Sara Nights,' a blonde, older, auxiliary nurse who spent most of her time turning me with the help of her colleague, The Bun Lady, a friendly women who was counting down the months to her retirement and always wore her greying hair in a knot on top of her head.

Outside the sisterhood of Saras was a collection of various nurses and auxiliaries who all has an impact on my life for a variety of reasons. Running Man, so-called because he was a fellow runner, was the wise man of the ward, a nurse with encyclopaedic knowledge, which I used later when I wanted to know how I could stop using nappies and catheter tubes.

There was 'Fussy nurse' who was in charge of health and safety, a camp male nurse who annoyed me as he took ages to hand out the drugs on the night round when I was trying to sleep, and Becky, a dizzy blonde who was on my wavelength. She was young and single and made me feel at ease in her care, I never felt embarrassed even when she had to change my nappies. The manager of the ward, Steven, was a jolly, larger-than-life character who liked to make staff and patients laugh. He would put on a silly accent and phone the ward, expecting the staff to fall for it, but they never did.

My rehab team included Sophie, a speech and language therapist, who later played an important role in preparing me to drink. Then there was Lucy, the occupational therapist whose early job it was to stimulate my muscles into working again. Lucy and I came to share a running joke that she did nothing, because I famously said to her that my progress was all my own doing and she thought that I thought she'd done nothing! My physiotherapist, Gemma, was a fellow runner who always believed I had the fighting spirit to run again and encouraged me along the way. There was also a young nutritionist who I later came to part company with because she was hell-bent on making me eat through the PEG in my stomach when I wanted to eat proper food. Looking after my emotional well-being was Lynne the psychologist. She was a gentle middle-aged woman who believed that meditation was the way forward. Lynne herself was in a wheelchair having been left paraplegic after a serious car accident many years before. She was an enormous help in the early days on the ward, acting as the go-between for my mum and Alison to voice their concerns about my medical care. But later her wheelchair became a barrier in our relationship. In my head I never wanted to be stuck in a wheelchair for life, so I felt I could not honestly share my feelings with her.

Ruling over all was my consultant neurologist, nicknamed Ming the Merciless, so-called because of his resemblance to the Flash Gordon baddie. What he said was the law and as he was always saying things that were contrary to what I wanted to hear, he could be very frustrating. He was the one who said I would never walk again, or even swallow.

But my favourite of all the Osborn 4 staff was Oliver, a forty-two-year-old father-of-two who had retrained as a nurse after working in customer services. He had the benefit of life experience on his side. Witty and passionate about music, over the months we shared many soundtracks to our lives and landmark moments.

Chapter 15
It's Like Shitting a Watermelon

LIFE ON THE REHAB ward was how I imagined it must be at boarding school – all rules and timetables to follow with no room for individuality. Many of the patients were in wheelchairs and every day they were pushed to the dining area at the centre of the ward for their meals, just like in a school canteen. And there they sat all day until their therapists came to wheel them off for their body-bending and tongue-twisting sessions. I was being fed via the PEG and avoided the mealtime routines but I had my therapy regime to follow like all the others.

Initially my physiotherapy was aimed at relieving the pain in my shoulders, which had been unbearable and I discovered was a common problem for people suffering from locked-in syndrome. My physiotherapist spent daily sessions with me, rocking my head from side to side to strengthen my neck muscles.

Every day I was hoisted out of bed and put in a chair. This was a grim spectacle for onlookers. Two nurses manhandled me enough to slide a sling under my body, which was attached to the mechanical hoist. As the machine started to lift my deadweight my body would flop in all directions: my head dangled to one side, my lifeless limbs dragged down by gravity. I looked and felt like a macabre and tangled puppet.

From my position in the chair I was hooked up to the FES machine (Functional Electric Stimulation) and my limbs would be shocked into twitching. Firstly my occupational therapy started with my right side, which had shown the initial flickers of movement. Electrodes were attached to my hand and for thirty minutes an electric current was channelled through my body to stimulate my muscles to contract and move. All the time I was watching, looking for movement and a sign that the pathways carrying messages from my brain to my muscles were being restored.

The electrical impulses shooting through my body took me back to April 6 1999 when I first came to understand the meaning of pain. I was pregnant with India, and having read all the National Childbirth Trust's advice for first-time mums I had opted for natural childbirth. I was given a TENS machine with an electrode on it attached to my spine. When I felt a contraction I had to press the switch and the electrical pulse was meant to intercept the pain signals to the brain and minimise the agony. After a twenty-five-hour agonising labour, India was born *au naturel*. A year later when I went into labour with Harvey I demanded the drugs straight away! On this basis, when Alison devised the pain chart for me in the ICU, she quite often asked me if the pain I was suffering compared to childbirth and if I blinked yes she knew she needed to get help immediately.

Three weeks after I arrived on the ward there was a breakthrough when I was given a buzzer. I still could not move my head or my arm but I had a tiny amount of movement in my right foot. Enough, they thought, to control a foot buzzer. What a contraption it was. The buzzer was placed on the pillow under my foot. I could not move my heel but with a short, juddery flicker of movement, I was able to hover the ball of my foot long enough to press the button to call for help. As you can imagine this turned out to be a recipe for disaster; with my limited control I was calling for help every few minutes, and it wasn't long before the nurses got fed up with my unintentional cries of wolf, so the buzzer was taken away. I thought back to a film Mark and I had watched many years ago about the artist Christy Brown who had cerebral palsy and learnt to paint and write with the only part of his body he could control: his left foot. How could a man create such beauty with just his foot when I could not even press a button?

One of the early goals for me and my therapists was 'static sitting' for three minutes; this is therapist-talk for sitting up. It sounds like a straightforward exercise but I had been lying on my back for six weeks and had no muscle control, so it turned out to be a huge challenge. Here I was introduced to the tilt table, a kind of plank on wheels which could be raised electronically. Whereas in the ICU I had been hoisted into a padded armchair that supported my lifeless body with lots of pillows in order to be taken into the garden, now my body was being trained to tolerate an upright position. I was hoisted out of bed and strapped onto this table. As the physios buckled the leather straps tightly around my limbs I was reminded of those American murderers who are sent to the electric chair. It made me feel like my life had become a death sentence in its own right. At first I was lifted to a half-horizontal position which was still enough to make the blood rush to my head and cause dizziness, so that I felt the ward spinning around me. Twice a week I was hoisted onto the 'Frankenstein table' until I was able to stay upright for several minutes at a time. In this 'standing' position I could feel muscles in my legs and ankles working again as they took my weight, at first they began to ache but gradually I got used to being in this position and my muscles grew stronger. I also liked being able to look people in the eye from an upright position rather than having them look down on me, it boosted my confidence. However this therapy was quite startling for my friends who occasionally had the misfortune of visiting during a tilt-table session and thought they had walked in on a crucifixion.

From this I advanced to sitting on the edge of the bed. Again this involved a tremendous amount of effort for both me and my therapists. I was hoisted into position with one arm on the bed, my feet would be positioned for balance and my therapists sat either side with another carer in front and behind. Gradually they moved away from me so that I was using my own strength to hold myself upright. As you can imagine this didn't always go to plan. At first I could feel myself falling. 'Tim-berrrr,' I could hear myself shouting in my head as I wobbled to the left then fell backwards. For one session Mark took the day off work so that he could watch my progress. 'That's brilliant, Kate,' he said encouragingly as he watched my therapists sit upright then move away as I held the position for a whole minute.

Another part of me that was also suffering from a lack of movement at this point was my bowels. I had often laughed at those cross-eyed women on TV commercials who shared the secrets of soft stools. Now I realised just how painful constipation was. It's fair to say it was up there with childbirth. For two weeks I suffered the most excruciating pain in my stomach. I had lost more than two stone and was being fed a high-calorie diet through the PEG to build up my weight, whether this was the reason for my constipation, I don't know. But the agony dragged me down.

One day my mum walked on to the ward and saw me in the corner of the ward, alone and in pain with tears rolling down my face. To make matters worse, the nurses on Osborn 4 were trying to wean me off the twenty-four-hour care I had been used to in the ICU, so were misinterpreting my tears as grief for my old life and therefore my tears went unnoticed. It was not a case of me being needy, I was bloody ill.

The stress and discomfort were so bad that I couldn't even face visitors. I was in constant fear of passing a movement in their company and having no control over my rear end just added to the pressure. I could imagine nothing more embarrassing that having a dirty nappy in company even if it was only Alison, Anita and Jaqui, who had all dealt with their fair share of pooey bottoms over the years. They arrived one afternoon having made the thirty-minute journey across the city to visit me, all chirpy and cheerful and ready to lift my spirits. But I had sunk so low, that was going to be impossible. I spelt out the words 'I'M SORRY YOU HAVE TO GO NOW'. Looking back I am ashamed at the way I behaved, it was rude. And while I may have been accused on many occasions of being short-tempered and impatient with the nurses, I would never have deliberately been rude to my friends. Once they had left I signalled to the nurses 'DO NOT LET ANYONE IN TO SEE ME'.

I was feeling low. At the worst I was having childbirth-like pain for twenty minutes at a time and then I would need to have my nappy changed. This was happening up to twelve times a day and I later found out that when I buzzed for attention, the nurses would play a game of paper, scissors, stone to determine which unfortunate one got the job. I hoped it would be 'Sara

Short' as I always felt comfortable in her hands. She never made a fuss; she just got on with the task as if it were the most normal thing in the world to change the nappy of a thirty-nine-year-old baby.

When I spelt out 'IT'S LIKE SHITTING A WATERMELON', she laughed and said 'Better out than in.' Up until that point she'd thought I was a posh girl because I came from Dore, but now she slowly glimpsed the real Kate.

At times when I was feeling depressed, and this was quite often in those early days of rehab, Alison would bring in her old photos to cheer me up. One of my favourites was a shot of Anita, Jaqui, Alison and I in our bikinis, lounging on the deck of a millionaire's yacht. Immediately I was lifted out of my miserable bed and transported to a vodka-laced afternoon in the Med sun in September 2009 when the four of us had gone on a long weekend to Spain with a group of ten mums from school. Jaqui and Anita had been on these girls-only breaks many times and always came back looking refreshed and tanned, with stories of kid and husband-free fun. It sounded like too good an opportunity to miss so Alison and I joined the party. On the day the photograph was taken we had been walking along the harbour, slightly merry from the afternoon cocktails, when we spotted what can only be described as a floating gin-palace. It was one of those boats that you wouldn't get much change from half a million pounds. Immaculate, white and gleaming, the sun glinting from its polished cherry deck caught our attention.

Champagne O'Clock was the name of the yacht and she certainly lived up to it. Fuelled by booze and bravado we walked up to the yacht and were invited on board by two German men with decent enough English. It seemed rude to turn down such an opportunity so Al,

Anita, Jaqui and I, and two other mums, hopped on for a couple of drinks. It turned out the German guys didn't own the boat– they had been asked on board by the owner, a middle-aged blonde woman from the Midlands, who was on her own while her husband was away on business. While we were all laughing and drinking on board Champagne O'Clock the husband arrived back and was sitting in a bar watching us having a party on his boat. Needless to say when he turned up on deck, he wasn't best pleased, but Alison charmed him and in no time he had invited us back the following day. As we left the yacht we arranged to return at noon the next day, giving the owners the option to set sail early if they changed their mind. Noon arrived and the other two mums got cold feet leaving just Anita, Jaqui, Alison and me to go through with our boat-crashing. As we walked down to the harbour, there was Champagne O'Clock and there were our hosts with the breakfast table laid and waiting. Croissants and orange juice followed; then more orange juice and vodka, then more vodka, then Pimms, then more vodka. The couple were the perfect hosts, they took us water-skiing and jet skiing and their staff waited on us hand and foot. For an afternoon we felt like we had joined the jet set. We had such a good time on that holiday that when I came home I was still buzzing, so much so that Mum accused me of having an affair because I seemed so happy. Charming, I thought.

Chapter 16
It's Just not PC to Say You're a Cripple

EVER SINCE I WAS hoisted into the padded support chair on wheels in the ICU I had loved being out in the fresh air. I would stare at the door that opened out on to the garden until whoever was at my bedside took the hint and called a nurse to get me strapped in, wrapped up and ready.

As I've said, I found my stare could be very effective. I remember an occasion when Alison and Anita were massaging my feet during one of their visits. In the early days this was a great comfort to me and Alison, being a hairdresser, was very good at it. Anita, on the other hand, was less forthcoming. She was caring and would do anything for me, but she hated feet and mine were particularly hideous with their twisted toes, curling yellow toenails and calloused skin. While Alison rubbed cream into my left foot, Anita strayed away and sat near my head. I could hear Alison asking her to come back and help with my feet, but Anita was resisting. 'Kate would rather I talked to her. Wouldn't you, Kate?' she asked. I stared at Anita, then looked down to my feet. Anita got the message and started massaging my right foot.

One afternoon I was sitting out in the garden with Mum when I stared at the communication chart, the sign that I wanted to say something. The route from my bed to the garden had passed by a plate-glass fire door and there, for the first time, I caught my reflection in the makeshift mirror. I didn't recognise the old woman I saw in the window. She was thin, her hair hung limp and grey around a face that was sallow and grey. Her eyes were sunken and hollow and her mouth gaped with a contorted scowl. I had aged thirty years. For more than three months I had managed to avoid looking in mirrors and now what I saw made my stomach churn. I saw the reason why my children always hesitated before they kissed me goodbye.

Mum picked up the communication board and starting reading through the colours. I blinked twice on red, the first line. Then she read through the letters on the first line …A? One blink for no. B? Again one blink. C? I blinked twice at C. Back to the beginning again. Red? Yellow? Blue? Green? Green I blinked twice on green. O? One blink. P? One blink. Q? One blink. R? Two blinks it was R. Moving to the blue line I blinked twice at the first letter I. Back down to the green line. I blinked twice on P. We repeated this for another P. Back to the start and I blinked twice on the blue line. I? One blink. J? One blink. K? One Blink. L? Two blinks. Back to the yellow line. E? First letter, two blinks. Finally I blinked twice to indicate the end of the word. CRIPPLE. There: I'd said it. I knew it wasn't politically correct, but there was no getting away from the facts. That's what I now was.

Mum threw the board down, saying, 'I'm not carrying on with it if you're going to talk like that.'

But I had only spelt out what I'd seen. It upset Mum to have me talk in such a way, but it was how I felt.

When I was alone my insecurities came back to haunt me. Did Mark see what I had seen in the reflection? Did he wonder what had happened to his Kate, the girl with the pretty hair and 'nice bum' that he had fallen in love with all those years ago? If he did, he managed to hide it well with a smile and a joke for me. But I couldn't help thinking that if I were in his shoes I would not want to spend the rest of my life with an invalid.

'WHY DID IT HAPPEN TO ME?' I spelled out one afternoon while Alison and Mum were sitting holding the board. I saw Alison flash a look at Mum as if to say, 'Shit! What do we tell her?'

Mum stepped in with the words of explanation that the Irish doctor had given her in those first couple of days. She said that sometimes it happened to people who were too fit. Super-fit people can push their blood vessels too far and clots occur. It appeared that was what I had experienced. I thought back to my life, and although it had not seemed excessive at the time, maybe I had been pushing myself too hard. The business start-up was putting me under enormous pressure to succeed, I had been pushing my body harder to become extra fit in order to take on the Kilimanjaro climb. With the personal training sessions and the military boot camps on top of my usual 70 miles a week running, I had been working out to the extreme. But I loved the challenge and exertion. In my head I set myself a goal. No way would I spend the rest of my life in a wheelchair, and I wanted to regain enough movement in my hand to point to the letters on the board or write down my thoughts, so I would no longer need to rely on the communication chart.

Chapter 17
They're Trying to Kill Me

FOR WEEKS AFTER MOVING to Osborn 4 I was haunted by an incident when I was convinced that one of the nurses in the ICU had tried to kill me. I wasn't sure if it had really happened or if the cocktail of drugs had caused me to hallucinate, but in my mind I was certain that the staff nurse on duty on the night in question had tried to terminate my life with a 'graphite' drip.

If I was being totally rational I should have realised that a 'graphite drip' does not exist and the nurse I thought had a death-wish for me was no longer caring for me, so, in effect, I was safe and should get over it. But a combination of being kept in the dark about my medical forecast in those early days, my own paranoia about being a case not worth saving, and the general boredom of being incapacitated, meant that I could not erase this incident from my mind. It was so vivid that in my head it had to have happened. And it kept playing over and over again.

I had tried to communicate this overpowering worry to Mark, who had the typical bloke's attitude that I should just get over it. My mum was more sympathetic when I tried telling her but was uncertain how to handle it without coming across as paranoid as her daughter. The whole incident was dragging me down and making me so depressed and upset that one afternoon during her visit Alison wheeled me out into the courtyard and asked in her usual matter-of-fact manner, 'What's the matter with you?' I could always rely on Alison to get straight to the point. Why pussyfoot around with feelings with your best friend? 'NURSE TRIED TO KILL ME,' I spelled out. I don't think she quite believed me.

'Is it bothering you?' she questioned me further. One blink for no.

'Are you worried that it will happen here?' Again I blinked once for no.

'Then why are you telling me? What do you want me to do about it?' Alison asked, using the tone of voice she normally adopted when her kids were giving her a hard time.

'SACK HER,' I blinked in reply as Alison burst into laughter, her warm, giggle always had a ripple effect in setting me off laughing like a naughty schoolgirl. And although no sound came from my mouth, my eyes started to smile for the first time in days.

Afterwards Alison and Mum exchanged notes and decided that as ridiculous as this episode sounded they could ignore it no longer. Mum contacted Lynne my psychologist and lodged a formal complaint. A senior sister was appointed to investigate. A meeting was set up with the complaints co-ordinator, a nursing sister, my psychologist, me and Mum. There we had the chance to explain about the whole 'graphite drip' incident and how the laughter and snatches of overheard conversations from the nurses who gossiped in the bay near my bed fuelled my paranoia. The nurse at the centre of the incident, when questioned, was upset by the complaint as she was under the impression that she had developed a good relationship with me. In fairness to her she was the one who started the whole communication process by making the laminated 'blink once for no, twice for yes' sign. But I always felt her caring side was a façade that went up when visitors were around and slipped when we were alone.

The real story behind my nightmare, it transpired, was that during the night in question my chest had deteriorated and I was suffering from sputum retention. The nurse attached a saline drip to the tube in my mouth to loosen the gunge on my lungs so that it could be sucked out more easily. I was also suffering from constipation and given a dark brown liquid laxative through my nose tube.

The investigation concluded: '*There is no indication of any drug or substance which could be classed as 'graphite'. We can reassure Kate that there was no intention to kill her with a 'graphite' infusion at any point in her stay.*

'It is common for ICU patients to have hallucinations, nightmares or false memories of their stay in the ICU. These fears can last for many weeks after discharge from the ICU. Patients also report feelings of paranoia and a few can have extreme symptoms of stress after their treatment in the ICU. These feelings can be helped by talking to a professional counsellor.

'The nurse conversations around the bed will be discussed at the critical care clinical and nurse management meetings. All the staff will be reminded of the importance of not participating in idle gossip in patient areas.

Three weeks later I had a follow-up visit from the investigating nurses. I had been using the communication board for several weeks and was in a position to communicate my concerns more eloquently through my psychologist who acted as my voice. Once again the nurses stressed that my poorly condition at the time could have been the cause of my delusional memory and I was embarrassed to admit that it was all probably a dream, but not a good Patrick-Duffy-in-the-shower-type dream. I still had concerns that I felt needed to be raised. I explained how I was very much aware that I nearly died and as a result was very scared. That fear of dying made me cry a lot, yet no one understood why I was crying, making me feel invisible and alone. I added that at times I felt the care wasn't great, no one explained to me what was happening and the staff always talked about me but never to me.

After a long and open discussion the nurses apologised for the 'failings in my care' and I was satisfied with their explanation. I just wanted to draw a line under the whole upsetting incident so that I could move on and decided against lodging a formal complaint. I was happy that the things that had been preying on my mind for so long were finally out in the open and I had answers. As a result of the investigation several shortcomings in the ICU care came to light and recommendations were made to pass on to all medical and nursing staff to ensure that:

1. All staff are aware of the importance of communication with the patient.

2. The patient gets constant reassurance.

3. The patient is made to feel safe at all times.

I felt that I had made my point and that something positive had happened.

Chapter 18
Don't You Dare Write Me Off

MY FIRST REVIEW ON Osborn 4 should have been a positive one. In the first month I had achieved some of my goals. I had managed to sit up with some help, I was being hoisted into a chair and I had proved that my mind was fully awake and able to communicate through the communication board. Considering I had been on the critical list, I thought I was doing OK. I knew I still had a long way to go but I was hoping for some good news when Mark, Mum, Alison, Ann and I met with my team of medics and therapists.

We gathered together in a side ward and Lynne my psychologist started off by telling of the 'conversations' we had via the letter board. I had told her that I wanted more physiotherapy and I was frustrated at being unable to get the nurses to come and attend me at night. My particular bugbear was Lorna, the night nurse. It seemed to me that whenever I blinked at her in an attempt to grab her attention, she deliberately turned her back and avoided me. Even when I was able to call for a nappy change using a buzzer, she was still the most unhelpful and would roll her eyes and say, 'in a minute'. I often wondered if she worked in a different time zone because her 'minute' was never less than half an hour. Although she was the worst, she wasn't the only one. There were other nurses who stuck their heads around the door when I buzzed for help and as soon as they could see I was breathing would walk away without checking what I needed, which annoyed the hell out of me.

My physiotherapist then explained how they were pleased with the results of my tilt-table exercises and that my right hand seemed to be getting stronger, although there was still no movement on my left side. It was all going well until Ming the Merciless suggested the therapists would need to visit our home.

'Why?' Mark asked in surprise. Ming explained that they needed to start thinking about my discharge from hospital and that they would need to look at what modifications and adaptations I would require for twenty-four-hour care back home in Dore. This was the first time there had been any suggestion I could leave hospital and I instantly perked up.

'But she can't come home. Look at her!' Mark replied defensively. His words hit me like a slap in the face. Suddenly the conversation had turned from being about my progress to me being a burden. To hear Mark rejecting me hurt so much. I wanted to scream out, 'I'm here and I still have feelings you know.' But it was too late, the emotional damage had been done in four little words 'She can't come home.' I wanted to die. If the one person who promised to stand by me in sickness and in health was turning his back on me where would I go? Maybe my insecurities were not all in my head. Inside my broken body, I broke down. Tears flooded down my face. In my head I was shouting, 'Damn you. Don't you dare write me off.'

I admit that at that point in time I was no catch for anyone. My feet were twisted, my head was propped up like a rag doll and there was a constant trail of dribble down the left side of my mouth. I had a catheter bag (without the matching shoes) and I was still being fed through the PEG in my stomach. None of the doctors, nurses or even my friends had mentioned the prospect of me going home. And even with all my optimism for a full recovery, I wasn't stupid enough to think I was ready to leave hospital.

I was devastated. I sat in my wheelchair, shaking with panic, thoughts racing through my head. What would happen to me? Where was my future? Mum and Alison, both shocked by what had happened, quickly wheeled me back to my bed. I stared at Alison, who realised I wanted to say something, and picked up the letter chart.

'STAND BY ME,' I blinked through watery eyes.

'Who are you talking to, me or your mum?' She was trying to be flippant, but I could hear a tremble in her voice. 'BOTH,' I blinked back as Mum took my flickering right hand in hers and Alison gave my lifeless left hand a reassuring squeeze, both fighting back their own tears. Kneeling down beside my wheelchair Mum said, 'All you have to do is make that flicker happen, make it work. Once you make those connections you will never lose the pathways in your brain.' Her words were all I needed to give me hope. I would work hard to make those connections. I would return to my home and my family.

This incident deeply affected Alison whose elderly father was in the best local nursing home in the area. She knew there was no way I could live the rest of my life in God's waiting room and would not allow it to happen. She relayed the incident back to Anita and Jaqui and they came up with an action plan. There was a new development of apartments being built on the outskirts of Dore. They would be expensive but they were modern and with a bit of work could be wheelchair-friendly. Between them they planned to cash some of their own investments and start fundraising with support of the Dore mums to secure me a home and pay for carers to look after me for the future. It was an ambitious plan but it made me realise the value of true friends.

The review had been a harsh reality check for all my family. Mum and Dave weighed up the possibility of me moving back in with them for the first time since I was seventeen. It would have meant great upheaval for them to sell up their home fifty miles away in Macclesfield and move somewhere close to my friends in Dore, but it was something they realised they might have to consider.

After the review, Dave went round to our house and had a serious man-chat with Mark. 'This is her home, her children are here and Kate needs to be here,' he stressed. Looking back I can now understand Mark's reaction. He was struggling to be a good father and a breadwinner, working long hours and juggling child care with his mum and my mum. To suddenly be told that he needed to think of adapting our home to make it wheelchair-friendly was the last thing on his mind at that point. He wasn't ready to contemplate a life as a full-time carer. He needed time to process such upheaval to all our lives. Neither Mark nor any of my family and friends had completely come to terms with the full extent of my ongoing dependency.

Following the review Mum spoke in private to Ming, who was deeply apologetic for the upset that had been caused. He accepted that the review was way too soon and should have focussed on the positive, albeit tiny, steps in my progress. He told Mum, 'You can never say never, but you have to be realistic with yourself. The chance that Kate will walk again is so remote. She may have some progress but you need to prepare yourself for the fact that she will depend on you.'

That night while my friends and family were dealing with the impact, I lay in bed and cried myself to sleep. I dreamt I was getting ready for my usual weekend run. I had my kit on, stuck two fingers up to Mark and ran. I was running free over the Peaks, both legs working, arms pumping and India, Harvey and Woody were running by my side. 'I don't need anyone to care for me,' I thought. 'I can look after myself. I will walk again.'

The next day when Alison came to visit I was a different person. As she said, I had got my spark back. Before the review the person she visited in the hospital bed wasn't Kate but an empty shell of a woman. She found it hard to imagine that even I could bounce back from such a fall. When mums at the school gates said inane things like 'she'll be fine,' or 'she'll be back on her feet in no time, just you see', Alison would often think, how can you say that, you haven't seen her? From that day onwards she saw Kate the fighter. Physically nothing had changed, I was still a cripple. But inside Mark's reaction had made me angry, and that anger had turned into a positive force which was driving me to make giant steps when all the medics were expecting were tiny flickers of movement. For me, getting better was no longer in the hands of the doctors, I was taking control.

Chapter 19
Hondas and Lawnmowers

UNTIL WE ARE FACED with a major trauma, none of us can really know how well we'll cope. And it was no different for Mark. Being the sort who would accept medical advice, he believed the doctors when they said I would never walk or talk again. He could see with his own eyes that I was a feeble imitation of the woman he had married, but he did not want to admit it to himself even though deep down he knew it to be the case. Furthermore he could not bear to tell any of his friends or work colleagues that I would never speak or run again. He carried the burden of acceptance alone and to keep himself from being sucked into depression he found escape in the most mundane blokey pastimes: car washing and lawn mowing.

Before the stroke Mark, like many men I would imagine, thought that families and homes ran themselves. He didn't realise what skills it took to be a supermum. The daily routine required diplomacy and discipline to prevent the potential disorder and chaos that inevitably comes with three children under the age of eleven. As he jetted off around the world on business trips to far-flung places like Chicago, Dubai and China, wining and dining doctors into buying his company's medical supplies, I kept the family together.

Now he was still going out to work, although he had cut back on the overseas trips so that he could be home at night for the children. At the end of the day he had the added stress of visiting me in hospital and trying to put on a brave face, which must have been harder than a day's work. By the time he arrived home, there would be chaos as Harvey or Woody had thrown a tantrum, refusing to be told what to do by their grandparents. Quite simply, Mark was running on empty.

So Mark often retreated to the garden shed, get out his lawn mower and cut the grass. Twenty minutes, every week and the satisfaction of a lawn as neat as Lord's Cricket Ground was his therapy. Personally I would have chosen a manicure or neck massage, but we are talking about Mark here and although he likes to think of himself as a modern, twenty-first century man, sometimes the twentieth-century behaviour slips out. My stepdad and Mark's dad regularly offered to mow the lawn for him. But no, this was his act of switching off, a time when all he needed to think about was keeping the Flymo in a straight line and not cutting the electric cable.

Sunday morning would be a similar routine. He'd get out the chamois leather and bucket and wash the car on the drive. In this Mark was no different to many of his friends. While he was washing the car many neighbours would stop to chat on their way to buy their morning newspapers – it gave him a sense of normality.

While I was still in the ICU and Mark had the power of attorney, he decided to sell my family car, a black Kia Sportage 4x4, and trade in his company Volvo to invest in his dream car, a black Honda CRV 4x4. The new car looked very similar to my old one, except that it was shiny and new and Mark's. In his head Mark had reasoned that he could not afford to keep my car on the drive while I was in hospital long-term. He needed a large family car that was reliable for his business miles and big enough for Dad's taxi service for the children. My car was in need of maintenance work, so it made economic sense to trade both in for the Honda. What he didn't realise was the message this act sent out to me, it said, 'Kate, you will never drive again.' That may be the reason he avoided telling me for some months. It was only one day while I was lying in my bed in Osborn 4 watching *Come Dine With Me* that he jangled his new Honda keys in front of me and admitted what he had done. I hated him for it and told him so with my eyes. I turned my eyes away from him in anger. Again it was Mark's actions that brought out the competitive streak in me. In my head I pictured myself driving through the country lanes of Dore in a red Mini convertible. Not only would I walk again, but I would drive again and Mark would buy me a new car, if he knew what was good for him.

Mountain biking was another of Mark's regular escapes. When I went out running I would use the time to reflect on the things that were stressing me out. The fresh air cleared my head and gave my mind space to breathe, too. Some of my best ideas for marketing would come from a morning run. But Mark was the opposite, for him riding his bike around the lanes of Dore was a way to clear his head of any thoughts. While I was in hospital Mark was surprised at just how easily he could sleep at night. By the time his head hit the pillow at 10 every night, he was so exhausted he would fall into a heavy sleep. No nightmares, no restless thoughts, just carefree slumbers until the following morning. Sometimes if he woke early he'd go out for a 5 a.m. mountain bike ride while the children and grandparents were still in bed and the world was still sleeping. By riding his bike he didn't have to lie there and dwell on his awful predicament. It was something he had always done and made him feel normal.

However this carefree cycling attitude did land him in hot water with one of the nurses on Osborn 4. During one of his Saturday afternoon visits Mark said, 'It's been a right hectic morning. India wanted me to chauffeur her down to Charlotte's so that Alison could take them to the cinema. Then I had to drop Woody off for his swimming lesson. And I had an hour to kill, so I took my bike out for a ride.'

'WHO WAS LOOKING AFTER HARVEY?' I blinked. 'No one,' came the reply. Once again Mark was treated to one of my 'withering looks'. He tried to mitigate the irresponsibility of his action by claiming, 'it was only for fifty minutes and Harvey said he would be OK on his own'. I started crying in anger, not just because Mark had been so irresponsible, but because I felt guilty. I should have been there to take care of Harvey instead of lying in a hospital bed watching *Saturday Kitchen*. Overhearing the conversation one of the nurses said to Mark, 'That was not the best thing to do.' Lesson learnt. Mark never left the children home alone again, or if he did he never told me.

Chapter 20
'You're not my Mum. I Hate You!'

IN THE NATURAL ORDER of family life, grandparents equal fun and treats. Homework, bedtime and school runs are not part of their remit. All those nasty rules are made by Mum and Dad. While I was so poorly in hospital and Mark was juggling work, home and visiting, it was left to both sets of grandparents to impose some sort of discipline, and my children didn't like it one bit.

Personally I'd have given anything to be at home, waiting at the school gates at home time, ferrying Woody to his piano lessons and packing sandwich boxes for the weekly swimming lessons. I looked forward to the family's Sunday afternoon visits while I was in rehab but it was no substitute for being home with them. Mentally their visits encouraged me to push harder to get better. I hated being an outsider, watching as others were forced to bring up my children. In the early days I had blocked out all talk of the children because it hurt too much, now I wanted to be at the centre of their lives again. I didn't want to be the Sunday afternoon disabled Mum any more. India, Harvey and Woody came on to the ward every week armed with paintings and home-made cards to add a splash of colour to my sterile bedside and their chatter would brighten my afternoon. They talked about school, Brownies, music, TV and football and I would spell out the things we could do together when I was better. They would also grumble about their grandparents.

India, Harvey and Woody loved their grandparents but they were no replacement for their mum and this led to many rebellions at home. Mark's parents were Grandma and Granddad who lived by the sea in Stockport. The children visited during school holidays and were spoiled rotten with trips to the beach and visits to the Splashworld water park. Similarly Nana (my mum) and Grandpa Dave were also associated with presents and fun. On the wall above the kitchen sink was the timetable I had written the morning of my stroke, it followed the usual full pattern. Call me a control freak, but there was a daily calendar for each of the children, myself and Mark. Time for reading and homework were charted alongside piano and dance classes for India, football training for Harvey and piano and swimming lessons for Woody. Even the meal times, visits from our cleaning lady, Mark's weekend bike rides and India's visits to friends for tea were all pencilled in. It was the only way I could keep up with the busy family schedule. Both sets of grandparents were under instruction from Mark to follow my timetable in order to maintain normality, and as weeks of grandparent rule turned to months, the children began to fight the routines.

I have already mentioned Harvey's dislike of Grandma's strange slippers on the stairs, but the resentment ran deeper and no matter how hard both sets of grandparents tried to do their best they never felt it was good enough. Anything and everything would spark a tantrum. Harvey's view was that it was nothing to do with his grandparents what he did, they were not his family. On one occasion Harvey decided he wanted to drink his bedtime milk out of one of our cut-glass brandy bowls, which had been a wedding gift. When Grandma Ann told him to be careful not to break it, he snapped, 'It's my house, I can do what I like.' Woody when forced to attend his weekly music classes would throw a fit and scream, 'I hate you, you're the worst grandma and granddad in the world.' If Granddad went to collect Woody from school he wanted Grandma to go. If Grandma went, he wanted Granddad. Of course what he really wanted was Mum. Nothing was right.

Even Grandpa Dave, usually so laid-back and placid, was pushed to breaking point by Harvey and his antics. One night he snapped and sent Harvey up to his room, as he stomped off up the stairs Harvey broke down in tears, crying, 'I want my mummy home.' How could Dave argue? They all did. Other times my mum would sit on the sofa giving Woody the hugs he was missing from me and she could feel him shaking. He'd cry, 'She will be home one day, won't she?' Nana Jan felt such a fraud replying, 'Yeah, but not yet.' In her mind she felt it would be a very long time, if ever, before I would be home to give Woody his hugs.

The most difficult thing for Mark's parents to handle was that they couldn't fix things. Mark was their only son. They were used to looking after him and making things right. A broken toy – Daddy would mend it. A scraped knee, Mummy would kiss it better. Lost things could be found. They were a shoulder to cry on, an ear to listen. Babysitters and money lenders, that's what they were, with no conditions. I remember when I returned to the UK after my travels in Australia, Mark had arranged to meet me at Heathrow airport. But on his way to the airport, the car skidded on black ice and crashed. One call to Daddy and things were fixed. His parents arranged transport to collect me from the airport and I was still able to get back to Sheffield in time for the rugby match that afternoon. It was all sorted, Mark didn't need to worry. Mummy and Daddy saved the day. But they couldn't fix what was going on around them now and felt like failures.

India had her own difficulties. Being the oldest and the only girl, she felt it was her job to step into my shoes. It was something she had always done. As soon as Woody was old enough to sit up in his cot, India had become his surrogate mother. She was only six years old, but when her baby brother woke up in the morning, she would take him out of his cot, give him his morning milk and sit with him in front of the TV, until Mum woke up. Practical and older than her years, that was what she did. Now she was eleven she felt that she didn't need anyone to look after her, she was capable of doing it all. She made tea for her brothers; she made sure Harvey's football kit was clean. She would walk Woody to his Beavers group in the village hall. It was true that she was very competent and caring and could do all these things. She thought she was capable of looking after her dad, and Mark agreed that she was an enormous support to him during these difficult times, but there still needed to be an adult running the show. As the strain began to show on India she would complain, 'I do everything here. Many times she phoned Alison in tears after fighting with Grandma, just so that she could hear a voice close to her Mum. India's physical health also began to suffer. She was complaining of sickness and stomach cramps involving several trips to the doctor's surgery with suspected irritable bowel syndrome, brought on by the stress. Despite Mark's best efforts to hold the family together, he was becoming more distant as he juggled work, hospital and home on a daily basis and the strain was showing on them all.

Mark's parents thought it would be a break to take the children away for a week, to give them some time out. Being semi-retired they had their twilight years sorted and liked their holidays, whether it was cruises or visits to their time-share in Spain. They had already cancelled two cruises because they felt unable to leave Mark on his own and now decided to book a caravan near Scarborough for the five of them for a week. It was be the longest week of their lives, they later said. The children couldn't settle, they wanted to be home. They were bored, they were used to playing games with Mum and Dad and at sixty-seven and sixty-nine Mark's parents just didn't have the energy to keep up with them. They were trying in their own way to deal with the situation, but it was hard. They didn't want to put any more pressure on Mark, who was retreating into his own world. They watched helplessly as the weight dropped off him and no matter what his mum cooked up for his tea he was always too exhausted or drained to eat it. As grandparents they could see the loving, kind and gentle relationship they had nurtured with their grandchildren was slipping away. The children noticed it too. Many times India or Harvey would ask, 'Why are you sighing, Grandma?' Mark's mum later compared the nine months to having a child. The pain of childbirth is unbearable at the time, but when you hold your baby for the first time, you forget the pain. When I came home, the pain was forgotten.

Looking back it was all understandable, the children were young, their mum had been snatched from them and they couldn't accept what was happening. But it still hurt those on the receiving end of the backlash.

Chapter 21
Proving Them All Wrong, Damn You!

WAS I IMAGINING IT or had my left thumb twitched? It was hard to tell whether it was an involuntary spasm or if my positive thinking was having an effect. Mark's reaction during my first review had made me more determined than ever to walk again. I had spent the night after the review in bed, staring at my thumb, willing it to flicker. Move, damn you, the words of frustration echoed inside my head. It was the same stubborn voice that used to push me to run that extra mile through the rain and the sleet high on the moors above Sheffield in the middle of winter when I wanted to give up. The one that says Kate, you know you can do it!

Move! I tried again. This time I could I could feel the tension throughout my body, but not so much as a twitch. If any of the nurses had seen me they might have thought I had slipped back into a coma and rushed me back to the ICU. At this point I had regained a minimal amount of movement in my right thumb and toe, but nothing on my left side. It was completely dead. Then it moved again. I was sure it was not my imagination. In my head it felt like I was giving a triumphant thumbs-up, but it was no more than a slight movement and certainly not enough to touch my fingers or hold a spoon. I did it again. This time it moved in time with my thoughts. I was controlling it. Was the physiotherapists' Functional Electric Stimulation working or was it the power of mind over matter? I couldn't be sure; anyhow I felt tired but satisfied.

The following day when Alison visited I waited until she was in the middle of one of her funny stories then I did it again. Alison stopped mid-sentence. 'Kate, did I just see your left thumb move?' I blinked nonchalantly as if to say, so what?

'That's amazing. Are you moving it all by yourself?' she asked, her eyes reflecting my own spark of pride. I was moving. From that moment my carers and I knew that my brain was forming new connections and where there was once a dead end, new pathways were opening up inside my head. I was reminded again of my mum's words of hope from the Irish doctor who said that the brain can form new pathways and I truly believed there was hope for me.

With every small but significant movement, my friends and family wanted to leap about and make a huge fuss, but they had to contain their excitement. They had been given such a bleak prognosis from the doctors that any small advance in my mobility was seen as incidental and not to be exaggerated for fear of raising my expectations. Mum and Alison would wait until they left the ward before giving each other the high-five in secret, like they were part of some shady sect. I later looked back at this time and questioned whether the doctors' and therapists' fear of giving false hope was just another way of being negative.

'You don't encourage our Kate,' is what my mum has said all my life. She knows me too well. I'm like a dog with a bone, never giving up. In my world rules are there to be broken; boundaries only exist to be pushed.

115

Sometimes Mark found this side of my character exasperating. When we were having our old kitchen converted into a new kitchen diner we often fought over the tiniest things. We had a £25,000 budget and Mark was determined not to overspend, on the other hand I wanted the best. Why scrimp on things like cheap five-pound door handles when you've spent so much on achieving quality? That was my theory. Guess who usually won?

With this limited movement to encourage me, I set myself new goals, always three or four weeks ahead of my therapists. Up until this point the therapy team had no experience of anyone with such a severe stroke regaining their movement. Even the advice from the National Institute of Neurological Disorder and Stroke said, 'while in rare cases some patients may regain certain functions, the chances for motor recovery are very limited'. There was little positive precedent for the therapists and me to follow. The most famous case of locked-in syndrome – Jean-Dominique Bauby, the French magazine editor on whose life the film *The Diving-Bell and the Butterfly* was based – never regained more than the ability to blink before his death. And stories of other cases on the internet and in the media rarely progressed beyond the blink of an eye or enough movement in one hand to operate a specialist computer or an electric wheelchair.

With this in mind I gave myself a new goal to be mobile enough to be able to join Mark and the kids on holiday at the start of June and pushed myself hard in therapy. My family also sat down with the team of therapists who mapped out an action plan. Top of my list of priorities was the removal of my tracheotomy or 'trachi' as the nurses fondly called it. In my mind the tube in my windpipe had only been a temporary

116

measure and I fully expected that one day it would be removed and the hole in my neck could start to heal. I was also desperate to start swallowing trials to check if I was able to drink Earl Grey tea once again. I still had the 'nil by mouth' sign above my bed and craved tea or any liquid to quench my desperate thirst. Both these actions had to be approved by a specialist doctor, and so began the first of many frustrating waiting games. Every morning I watched as he made his rounds, hoping that today would be the day he'd allow the tests to begin.

Eventually the specialist doctor examined my breathing. He put his hand over the end of my trachi cap to test whether I could breathe without artificial help and when I passed this simple test he agreed that I could be put on a SATS machine, or oxygen saturation monitor. A clip was attached to my toe which monitored the percentage of oxygen-rich haemoglobin molecules in my blood. By shooting a pulse of light through my toe, the machine was able to work out the percentage of oxygen in my blood. The machine was alarmed and if my oxygen level dipped below eighty-nine per cent it would start beeping like a microwave oven. I could only have the trachi taken out if I could manage forty-eight hours without setting off the alarm. For the next few days I became obsessed by that bloody machine, it became like Woody's Operation game, where an unsteady hand created a buzz and meant you lost, but instead of picking bits of plastic body parts out of a board with a tweezer, my game of skill required nothing more complex than filling my lungs with air on my own, yet I couldn't quite manage it. I'd feel my breath getting shallower and watch the reading on the monitor start to plummet but no matter how hard I tried I couldn't stop it buzzing. This became particularly frustrating as I crept closer to the forty-eight hour cut off point and would have to start all over again. Once I blinked to Alison to take the probe off my toe. When the nurse saw what she'd done she gave her a row, stressing how important it was to monitor my breathing. 'It was her fault, she told me to do it,' said Alison, pointing at me as I lay helpless in my bed wearing the most innocent expression I could manage. I was delighted when I finally passed the test but the excitement was short-lived. Like everything in hospital, I discovered you have to wait for the doctor and my doctor was not due for another three days, so began another waiting game. When he eventually came back on the ward it took him all of two minutes to pull out the trachi tube and seal the cap.

In the days that followed I suffered a serious chest infection, which worried both my carers and the nursing staff. By day two my chest was rattling and I was gasping for breath like a hundred-a-day smoker. There was fluid on my lungs and I felt as if I was drowning in my own bed. I still could not cough so a machine was brought in to help me 'cough'. This was a particularly unpleasant experience and did nothing to alleviate the feeling of drowning as air was violently pumped into my lungs using a sealed mask over my nose and mouth. The idea was that once the air was in my lungs it would loosen the fluid allowing the 'lung hoover', which I had first encountered when I had been allowed sips of Earl Grey tea in the ICU, to suck it out. I was on heavy-duty intravenous antibiotics to clear the infection but the major fear for everyone, myself included, was that the infection would turn to pneumonia. I later found out that I was so ill the medical team had asked my physiotherapist to stay on duty all over that weekend so she could massage my lungs to help loosen the fluid. They were seriously worried they would have to reinsert

118

the trachi, I was seriously worried that I might die. After many uncomfortable days, my condition stabilised. But it was still an unpleasant time, especially for Mark. As the one closest to me, he often found himself on the receiving end of my impromptu expulsions. It was strange that even though I could not cough of my own accord I had involuntary splutters and without warning the gunge would come out, like a baby being sick. I will never forget the look of disgust on his face when he leaned over to kiss me and I vomited chest slime all over his new tie.

'Thanks Kate, nice to see you too,' he joked as he wiped mucus off his best work suit.

Once the drama of the chest infection was over, I was assessed for speech and swallowing exercises. My chest secretions were still being monitored but I was keen to start drinking again. 'You've got very weak lips,' my speech and language therapist Sophie told me after asking me to stick out my tongue as part of my first assessment. Blimey! That's got to be a first, I sniggered to myself as I recalled the glazed expression that Mark would adopt, which generally meant that I had been talking for too long and he had stopped listening half an hour ago. Sophie had asked me to stick my tongue out, which in theory seemed like a pretty simple request. A poke of the tongue indicated defiance and I was good at that, just ask my mum. However when I tried to stick my tongue out for Sophie it took every ounce of strength in my body just to part my lips a fraction, there was a flicker of the tip and nothing more. I was more exhausted than I would have been running across the fells. But it gave me hope. I could feel my tongue pressing against the roof of my mouth, that had to be a good sign for the future?

I was given a series of 'tongue-base strengthening

exercises' to work on with my therapists and carers. I had to do things like smiling with my mouth shut to activate the muscles in my mouth; stick my tongue out as far as I could, keep it flat and hold it there for a few seconds then pull it back in as far as I could. I had to repeat both exercises five times; then I was told to hold my tongue between my front teeth and swallow while still keeping my tongue tip between my teeth. This was trickier. And for the finale I had to poke my tongue out and waggle it from the left to right, holding for a few seconds at either side. The fit Kate inside my head was telling me this was a pretty pathetic exercise regime. When I was alone in bed I practised these exercises over and over again. My therapist suggested that I should use a mirror but initially I refused. At that time I had not seen my reflection, apart from in the plate glass door, but I could imagine how bad I looked and I didn't want to be confronted with it. Instead I waited until my visitors arrived and practised for them. 'Well done, Kate. You're doing great,' they would all say. It was only some weeks later when I had mastered the art of tongue-waggling that they admitted it hadn't even flickered, they had just been humouring me.

Another exercise designed to improve the strength of my cheeks and soft palate involved a ping-pong ball. Holding a straw in my lips, I had to blow a ping pong ball across the table, like a game of blow football. I had to repeat the exercise both when holding my nose and without holding my nose in order to feel the air pressure building up in my mouth. But the only pressure I ever felt building up was the need to giggle, particularly when the speech therapy assistant who I nicknamed 'Go Ape Girl' was in charge. I called her 'Go Ape' because she worked at the Go Ape climbing centre in Sherwood Forest at the weekends. She was lively and full of energy and always brought out my mischievous side. I couldn't help thinking about my mad months in Thailand and the lurid ping-pong sex shows advertised in the strip clubs of the Patpong District, so I found it hard to concentrate on my own rather less inspiring ping-pong exercises without laughing.

As the weeks passed I finally perfected sitting on the edge of the bed with no help and the therapy team was at last able to move on to 'dynamic tasks'. Now these probably sound more adventurous than they were. 'Dynamic' was therapy-speak for turning my head and reaching out with my right arm while sitting up.

When all my daily therapy sessions were over I'd practise on my own in bed or with the help of my carers until I was exhausted. This did not always please my therapists. One time when I was lying alone in bed watching TV I discovered I could lift my back off the mattress at will. This was great and I practised for hours. However my therapist found out and warned me to stop. My neck muscles were doing all the lifting work and not my core muscles, she said. So while I thought I was exercising the muscles that would help my balance and eventually help me stand up, all I was achieving was neck muscles like a Russian shot-putter. Initially I wouldn't accept the therapist's advice, thinking I knew my body better and continued flexing my back whenever I could. Then one day my therapist came in with a photograph of a female bodybuilder with a neck like a Rottweiler, which she pinned to my locker with the words *Do you want to look like this?* written above it. Point made, I stopped.

Alison later told me about a conversation she had with my physiotherapist around this time when I was pushing myself as hard as I could. My therapist said, 'The trouble with Kate is that her goals are too high.' To which Alison replied, 'But that's Kate. She was a real driving force before the stroke. Maybe you experts should meet her halfway.'

Chapter 22
The Whole Community's Involved Now

GRID 2 WAS A specialist computer and software package which allowed patients with no speech and limited movement to write text and 'speak' with an electronic computer-generated voice which was activated by a switch. When I started moving my right thumb, the therapists told my family that I might benefit from this equipment. In my head I had already decided that walking was more important to me than talking, but if there was a chance of having both then I wanted it all. I had been assessed by my therapists and it was considered suitable for my needs.

Within days my therapists had borrowed one from another department and it was duly set up next to my bed with the screen in front of me. The switch in my hand gave me a new freedom, whereas I was still not strong enough to hold a pen or write, I could move the on-screen cursor with slow, juddering actions to spell out words, press the alarm button to call for help and even channel hop on the TV. As soon as I was left on my own I started to experiment in using the screen to spell out words. Using the alarm, I called Oliver, my favourite nurse. As he walked towards my bed, he noticed I was looking rather satisfied with myself. On the screen I had typed the words I WILL WALK

AGAIN. 'Yeah, right,' he laughed. I remember the date vividly: May 1 2010. No one really believed those words, except me. It was my mantra.

The only problem with the GRID 2 computer and software package was the cost: £6,000. My friends wanted to help me to 'talk'. I suspect they were probably getting bored with the hit-and-miss communication board too. Anyway whatever their motives they put their heads together over a glass of Shiraz and came up with a plan to organise a charity event to bring in some cash.

Dore's network of villagers, school mums and dads and church members was constantly offering money to Mark to show their support. They had already been kind enough to cook for the family, which Mark had gratefully accepted. But money was different and, uncomfortable with the idea that our family should be treated like a charity case, he flatly refused to accept their donations. He was working, bringing in a decent wage, and I was being treated on the NHS so there was no need for handouts, no matter how well-meaning. Yet the offers kept coming and it was Anita, Alison and Jaqui who hatched the plan for a charity bike ride.

At first Mark took some convincing but eventually he caved in under pressure and agreed to organise a low-key sponsored bike ride for the children and their friends around one of the local beauty spots, Ladybower and Derwent Reservoirs. None of them had any idea how to organise an event. That was my job. I was the one who could 'persuade' people to do extreme things for a good cause. I had already successfully completed the Three Peaks Challenges for charity and I had come up with the idea to climb Kilimanjaro in aid of a local children's hospice. And I would have loved to be cycling around the reservoirs on a sunny spring afternoon rather being hoisted around the ward.

The reservoirs reminded me of a mad afternoon with Mark when we were first dating. We had cycled out for a picnic. When we arrived we were hot and sticky and in need of refreshment. Ignoring the 'Danger! No Swimming' signs we dared one another to dive-bomb into the water. I jumped first and Mark followed. It was bloody freezing. How we didn't die of heart attacks from the shock to our bodies I don't know. But it didn't stop us doing it again and again, until we were exhausted and exhilarated.

With the date and venue set, the charity bike ride took on a life of its own. Perhaps I helped subconsciously by willing my children and friends to make it a success that would make me proud. And they did. On the day more than 200 people turned up and cycled the twelve-mile route around the perimeter of the reservoirs. Harvey showed he was his mother's son by racing off ahead of everyone and finishing first. India completed the route at a more sedate pace with her girlfriends and even Woody managed a good distance, until he threw his bike down in a strop just two miles before the finish line and Mark had to remind him that he could either walk back and take at least an hour or cycle back in a fraction of the time.

When the ride was over, all the participants rested their sore bottoms and had a picnic by the side of the reservoir. The children played together, the grown-ups laughed together and Anita later said it was one of those perfect afternoons where there was a real feeling of camaraderie. There was just one shadow over the event – me. It sounded like the kind of afternoon I would have loved to be at the centre of. I was in spirit and in image. Mark had produced a six-foot-long Kate's Bike Ride banner with a huge photo of me which hung over the start and finishing line. As each person completed the course they signed the banner. When Mark brought it in to hospital later that evening he was still buzzing from the thrill of their success.

'I know I was reluctant at first, but there was a great sense of community spirit and everyone there had a great time,' Mark gushed. 'Even my boss and his wife turned up with a basket of home-made cakes and shared them out. The children's headmistress fell off her bike and embarrassed herself in front of everyone, we had such a laugh. I only wish you had been there Kate. We've raised £10,000, so we can order your new computer and get you talking.'

With the order placed, I would just have to wait a few weeks for it to be delivered.

Chapter 23
Visitors are Like Buses

MY FULL PROGRAMME OF therapy meant that quite often my visitors would have to wait in line to see me. Every day there was an hour of physiotherapy, an hour of occupational therapy and two hours of speech therapy; quite often my sessions overran the start of visiting hours. Without fail Alison or Anita would turn up at 2 p.m. but their visits were always restricted to forty minutes as they had to leave to pick the children up from school. I became quite the expert at keeping time for my visitors, making sure they left on time even though I wished they could stay longer.

Some days visitors arrived like buses, three or four at a time, when the limit was two to a bed. Other times there were none at all, which made for lonely afternoons. Alison devised a visiting rota, which she stuck on my locker so that I knew where I was and who I would be seeing. Initially when I was still very poorly this was restricted to just my close friends and family but, as I improved, the Monday to Friday slots were filled with various Dore mums, who would meet up in the car park and fight over the limited parking spaces. Evenings were times for family with Mark, his parents and my mum spread out over the week. And Sunday afternoons were reserved for the children and Mark.

During these visits the children became more comfortable around me and would take it in turns to sit near my face and mop my brow with cotton wool and Simple toner. I looked forward to these moments of intimacy with them.

To ensure I didn't miss out on any gossip during the restricted visiting period, Alison came up with the idea that friends in the village who wanted to show their care and support should write letters. She would them read them out to me, which not only gave her a new topic of conversation but made me feel like I was still a part of their busy lives.

My favourite of all the letter-writers was Anna of the fish-pie fame. Sensible, stoic Anna always managed to channel her dry wit on to paper and with four kids she had a constant supply of news. But the letter that amused me was the story of celebrity Katie Price. I had missed out on the most exciting bit of gossip to hit Dore in years – the serial bride formerly known as Jordan was buying a house in Dore Road, which was just up the road from where we lived. At the time she was making headlines for her marriage to the cross-dressing cage fighter Alex Reid.

Anna wrote *I can't imagine why she wants a house in Dore but hey won't it be funny bumping into her in the Co-op. Titty envy will be on the up in the village. Padded bras, chicken fillets and pink tracksuit, can you imagine it?*

I couldn't. Her letter continued*: I won't mind bumping into that new husband of hers, Alex. I'll be his paper girl any day.* It later transpired that the Chinese whisper had been wrong; Katie Price was actually buying a horse in Dore.

Other letters came from Amy, who ran the nursery in Dore which all my children had attended, and Sharon, whose daughter was my babysitter. I particularly looked forward to getting Sharon's reports as her crude and sarcastic sense of humour always shone through and Alison had to lower her voice when reading them out, so as not to offend any patients in the neighbouring beds. In time, as my recovery progressed and I felt ready to see more people, Amy, Sharon and another friend Kerry would be my company for a Monday night girlie night-in. They spent a couple of hours around my bed, chatting and gossiping like old times, reminding me of what life could be like again.

After the mums left, time dragged until 6 p.m. when Mark or his mum and dad or my mum and Dave would visit. This was the time that I became a connoisseur of TV cookery shows. *Masterchef*, *Come Dine With Me*, *Ready Steady Cook*. I loved them all. The highlight of my day was the *Great British Menu* at 5 p.m., which was ironic considering I had not been able to eat for months and was being force-fed liquids through the PEG in my stomach. I loved watching as top chefs from all over Britain competed to create a celebration dish. In the early days I had to depend on the nurses to switch the TV channels for me. Mark would bring in a TV guide and highlight my favourite programmes, but this was generally ignored. So imagine my delight when I regained movement in my thumb and I could channel hop using the thumb switch, which gave me control of my viewing choices.

The doctors had always told Mark to expect permanent brain damage, but it finally hit home one day when he walked onto the ward and caught me watching *The Jeremy Kyle Show*. In my old life I wouldn't have been caught dead watching a succession of chavs fighting over paternity tests and trying to cheat the lie detector.

But my concentration was so poor that mindless programmes were all I could manage to focus on and it's surprising how quickly the time passes when you need to know the answer to the all-important question, 'Did you sleep with my best friend?'

If I could catch the nurses' attention they would switch on my iPod and speakers and I could pass away some time listening to eighties and nineties indie music. Music is a powerful tool for stimulating the memory, which is why they use it in therapy for many Alzheimer's sufferers. In those iPod hours the songs of the Stone Roses, Happy Mondays, Inspiral Carpets and others would take me back to the hedonistic days of the Madchester music scene and our wild nights out at Manchester's Hacienda club. One song that always seemed to be played on a loop was The Smiths' 'Bigmouth Strikes Again', which to anyone who knew the old Kate was quite appropriate. I often wondered if the nurses were trying to tell me something.

I was also treated to several beauty therapy sessions from Mark's sister Jo, whose name was on the rota. Mark's family called us 'the Twinners' because we had a habit of turning up for family events wearing exactly the same clothes. We had always had an almost psychic connection and our friendship went way back to the rugby club days in Sheffield. Jo knew that I would not stand for hairy legs and bushy eyebrows. Unfortunately rehab was no beauty salon and Jo knew that under normal circumstances I would be embarrassed to be seen with just a couple of days' stubble on my legs. After all that time in the ICU my legs were looking like a sheepdog and my eyebrows were starting to resemble Noel Gallagher's, so Jo turned up with her beauty bag of tricks, a disposable razor and tweezers, and restored my dignity.

As I watched Jo go to work on my hairy legs, she talked about her life: the new house she and her husband had bought as a renovation project, and how well her oldest son Henry was doing at school. I have always had a soft spot for Henry, who is five months older than India, and from Jo's previous relationship. I was reminded of a conversation we'd had just a few weeks before the stroke. It was late one night after Christmas, we'd had several glasses of red wine and the talk had turned to morbid life and death what-ifs. It seemed quite prophetic in light of what happened next, but I asked her if anything happened to me would she look after my children. Naturally she said yes. In turn I promised that if anything should happen to her I would take care of her three children. I wondered if Jo was thinking what I was thinking, how it had all been a close shave.

It seems quite trivial to be talking about hair removal and toe-nail painting given the circumstances, but these, along with regular foot and hand massages, were all small acts of kindness that my visitors felt they could do without getting in the way. And it also brought us closer, particularly in the case of my half-sister Abi. We had never been close growing up as I was fourteen years older, and a rebellious teenager when she was born, and by the time she was four I had left for America. She was now living forty miles away in Manchester and making a career in television film-making, working on a BBC daytime drama. But once a week she took time out of her busy schedule to visit me. She would bring a selection of nail polish and allow me to choose the colour before painting my nails. This might seem like a small gesture but one that gave me a feeling of self-worth. While she was painting my nails she would talk to me about the drama that went on behind the scenes on the set of the TV show she was working on, which

131

made a welcome change from watching TV.

When my visitors had left and I was alone, I had time to reflect on their busy lives and the contrast with my own therapy-obsessed world. One thing that none of my friends had mentioned was Mount Kilimanjaro, even though it had been the one thing I hadn't stopped talking about before the stroke. Maybe they were being polite and didn't want to remind me of another thing I had lost, but I was interested to know if it was still going ahead. We had all paid our £300 deposit in January and the final instalment of £1,600 was due. One evening in June, Anita, Jaqui and I were sitting out in the garden in the dimming light when I stared at the communication board which Anita had let drop down by the side of her seat. I started to blink the message 'I'M SORRY ABOUT KILI'. It put the sore subject back on the agenda as a topic of discussion. Jaqui confessed that I had been the reason she was making the trip and without me there was no reason to go. 'Maybe another time,' I blinked through sad eyes. Deep down we all knew that wasn't going to happen.

Chapter 24
Facebook Saved my Life

THERE WAS A SIGN attached to the computer at the nurse's station on Osborn 4 which read 'Facebook is prohibited. Any staff found using it will be disciplined.' Like many workplaces the social network was out of bounds for the caring profession. I could imagine how frustrated I would have been if I was waiting for pain relief and the nurses were updating their Facebook status, but for me it was an essential tool of my trade. As a digital marketer, Facebook was my primary means of communication; in an age where so many people are addicted to their smart phones, it is the way to do business. Setting up new pages for my clients, sending out invitations to events, breaking news of special offers, Facebook was my professional lifeline. I had an idea. As I was unable to talk, Facebook could be my voice.

When Mark came in to visit me one night, I used the switch and the specialist GRID 2 computer beside my bed to spell out 'ask nurse can I use computer'. 'Why?' Mark questioned. 'Want internet,' I replied. The bedside computer had its uses for writing but it wasn't connected to the internet. Mark went off in search of Running Man, and came back with the answer I wanted. When the time came to say goodnight, Mark wheeled me out to the nurses' station and left me in front of the computer screen.

'You do realise I could get into serious trouble if I'm caught allowing you to use my Facebook account,' Running Man warned. 'But as you're a fellow runner, I'll take the risk,' he joked as he tapped his name and password into the computer and I was away. My left hand was still only flickering, but I had enough movement in my right arm, which was propped up on a cushion, to hold the mouse and click my way to a new lifeline.

I logged on to my account. My last post had been on January 31, exactly one week before the stroke. I had asked my generous friends to support me in my Kilimanjaro adventure and help raise cash for the Bluebell Wood Children's Hospice. The words seemed fresh in my mind yet Kili was now a challenge too far. As I started to update my profile with my shaky hand, I thought how far I had already come.

I wrote:

Hello, I thought you might be interested my story. On February 7 2010 I unfortunately suffered a major stroke. My survival chances were 50/50 and it was utterly devastating. Not normal for a fit 40-year-old mum of three young children, but an awful blood clot to my brain stem which caused me to become paralysed with locked-in syndrome. I used to road run, such as the Sheffield half marathon 1 hr 35 min then I moved on to fell running around 12 miles at a time. Imagine being buried alive, only able to blink…? While I wanted to die in the ICU, I'm glad I didn't now.

Seeing the words on the screen fired me up as I went on to catalogue the events following the stroke.

I wasn't given much hope. I'm still in hospital. My husband and family have been amazing as have the staff on my rehabilitation ward. I am very determined and motivated anyway and I want to prove wrong the people who have written me off! I've also been lucky in that I've had the most amazingly supportive family and friends, notably Mark, Alison and Anita, and my mum and Dave. I hope I am able to make a full recovery, the way I see it I have no choice but to get properly better.

That was it, I had said it. It had taken me more than an hour to write those few words, but the experience was liberating. Next I decided I'd send a message to my old friend from university, Cheryl. The last time I had seen her was the previous summer. She was now living out in Dubai with her husband and kids but we kept in touch via Facebook, exchanging embarrassing bad-hair photos and reminiscing about our university days almost twenty years before.

I typed:

Hello Cheryl. Have you heard I've had a stroke. Still in hospital. I was locked in, but I will walk and talk again.

Bloody hell, her stunned reply came back from 3,000 miles away. She'd had no idea what had happened. I guess that updating my Facebook page had been low on the list of priorities when I was fighting for my life. We were now able to communicate and her words of encouragement from far away boosted my determination.

After my first Facebook conversation I was addicted. Every day I wanted to be wheeled out to the nurse's station for a virtual chat with all my old friends. Some nurses were more accommodating than others. The friendly ones were happy to log me on and leave me in front of the screen while they carried on with their work on the ward. I was regularly to be found at the nurse's station when my visitors started arriving in the evening. When my therapists turned up for my daily sessions and found an empty bed, they knew where to look. However there were one or two who didn't approve and refused to let me loose on their work station. The downside of this addiction was the red sores I developed on my arm from where I sat typing for hours at a time, the skin becoming raw as my only working limb rubbed against the pillow beneath it.

I was reconnecting with my old life via the internet, poking people I had not spoken to in years and updating my friends on my daily routine. Facebook become my mouthpiece and my digital record of progress. In the days leading up to the charity bike ride on May 23 I posted:

Thank you everybody for your support. I am keeping my fingers crossed it keeps dry.

As my mobility improved I posted encouraging updates on my progress and when things were not going fast enough for me I would use Facebook as an outlet for my frustrations with messages. On days when my occupational therapist asked me to exercise my fingers by squishing a ball of putty in my hand, I later used my fingers to write:

Why is playing with putty so dull?

At other times when I was frustrated that therapy wasn't moving ahead fast enough for my liking, I wrote:

Fed up with my life. Why doesn't anyone get this?

I knew that there would always be a friend on the other end of my messages with words of support and empathy and this gave me an enormous boost when I was down. When things were going well it also gave me a greater sense of achievement to share it with a wider audience and get an instant reaction.

As well as being my lifeline, my computer also became a great bonding tool with some of the nurses. There was one auxiliary nurse in particular, who would find excuses to attend to my needs thanks to my laptop. When I was moved into a private room she quite often sneaked in and used my laptop to access her Facebook account, which was banned in working hours. It was our secret and it meant that I got special treatment as her favourite patient.

Chapter 25
Retail Therapy and Grey Roots

'I'M NOT GOING SHOPPING with you looking like a badger,' Alison announced one day as we were making plans for a pre-fortieth birthday spending spree. Meadowhall Shopping Centre was just a short taxi ride away from the hospital. Built on the site of a former steel works, with 280 shops under one roof and wheelchair-friendly access, it was just the place to start a programme of retail therapy. Staff at Osborn 4 encouraged patients to go there when they were ready for day trips. I had already spelled out to Alison that we should go to Meadowhall for coffee as soon as I was able to drink again. In my old life, when I worked as marketing manager for a company which owned thirteen restaurants at Meadowhall, I was a frequent visitor to the centre and was looking forward to getting out and about. For my birthday Mark's parents wanted to buy me a watch so Alison and Mum decided we should hit the shops and spend, spend, spend.

Before we could go, there was the small matter of my roots. Being a hairdresser, Alison was a stickler for covering up my signs of grey. Underneath my copper-brown, shoulder-length hair I was completely grey, but thanks to my six-weekly colouring sessions with Alison I had always managed to keep it under wraps. Three months had passed since my last hair appointment. My hair had grown wiry, dry and grey but I really didn't care what I looked like. I just couldn't be arsed with all the fuss. I knew I looked like crap and it would take more than a pot of copper colour to make the transformation. While my chest had been bad I had an excuse: the nurses thought the ammonia smell from the hair dye would affect my chest. Now there was no excuse and Alison wasn't going to let it go.

'There's no point,' I protested. But Alison had got clearance from the nurses and turned up on the ward one morning before the bath and shower routine with her crimper's bag of tricks and Anita as her assistant. She proceeded to mix up the colour and apply it as best she could to the bit of my head that was on show while I was lying down and in no physical state to fight back. The nurses then hoisted me out of bed and onto the plastic shower bed and I was wheeled into the shower room, stripped and had the colour washed off my hair.

I remember thinking it was all too much trouble to be stripped and showered just to have my hair dyed, but Alison insisted.

Deep down I was quite looking forward to my shopping trip; there was still a part of the old Kate that wanted to get out and have fun, and an afternoon in shopping heaven was a step in the right direction. I was also apprehensive. For four months I had not been outside the hospital regime of therapy, bed baths, doctors, nurses and visitors. I was comfortable in a world where everyone around me had something wrong with them and I wasn't ready for going out in my current state. I was dribbling constantly, I was strapped into a wheelchair with my head held in place and my arms supported on pillows and I looked like I felt – a mess.

On the big day, two of the nurses, Sara Bob and Sara Short, escorted me on my journey in the back of a specially adapted taxi while Mum, Alison and Anita followed by car. Once we arrived at the centre, the Saras melted into the background allowing Mum and my friends to take me around the shops.

Concerned for my psychological welfare, Alison and Mum had come up with a plan to protect me should we meet someone who was seeing Stroke Kate for the first time. In their grand scheme they would whisk me away in the opposite direction so that I wouldn't shock the person – and, more importantly, I wouldn't be upset by their reaction.

Everything was going fine as I was wheeled from one jeweller's to the next, browsing trays of expensive watches. The in-laws had been generous, and with a budget of £500 I had plenty to choose from. A White Ice watch with a big white face caught my eye and everyone liked it. When Alison looked at the price tag of £60 I said via my communication board 'NO. GOT MORE TO SPEND.' So our search continued until I found a Gucci watch which I really loved with a price tag of £650. 'It's too expensive,' Mum warned but Alison could see the hungry look in my eyes and suggested that Mark might be happy to make up the shortfall if we asked. While she went outside the shop to call him, we waited at the counter. I could imagine Mark's reaction on the other end of the phone. He always despaired when I went shopping. If he said I could spend £50 on a new dress, I would come back with one for £100. If he told me we could afford one pair of new shoes, I'd come back with two. I was smirking to myself when my mood changed dramatically.

A woman I recognised from my old gym walked into

the shop and without thinking uttered the words, 'Oh my God, what's happened to you!' Up until this point I had been surrounded by close family who had shielded me from the reality of how poorly I looked but this woman was just saying what they had all thought at some point. Her words stung me, but the real killer was the expression on her face, a mixture of horror and pity. Her reaction was no worse than my own when I had first spotted my reflection in the glass hospital door. But it came from someone who only knew me as the woman who spent hours pounding on the treadmill and so it really hit home how incapacitated I was. Unable to hold back the tears, I cried uncontrollably. The woman realised how insensitive her words had been and began to apologise, it upset her to see me in pieces. We must have looked a sight, her stammering and trembling, me wailing like a fog-horn and Anita trying to calm everyone down. At that moment Alison walked back into the shop, took one look at me in tears and put her avoidance plan into action. In a move worthy of Lewis Hamilton, she took control of the wheelchair and whizzed me out of the shop. I'm sure I could smell burning rubber as the wheelchair tyres turned.

Outside she looked at me and, with a wicked glint in her eye, said, 'What are you crying about? I've got the extra money.' She was delighted that her powers of persuasion had squeezed the extra cash out of Mark and her effervescence lifted me out of my self-pity. Leaving Anita to console the gym woman, Alison took me back to the jeweller's and I bought the watch. I had faced another obstacle and dealt with it. I have no doubt that the poor woman felt as awful as I did but it gave me strength to face other passing acquaintances, although I never got used to being stuck in my 'invalid chariot' and vowed that as soon as I was up again I would walk.

141

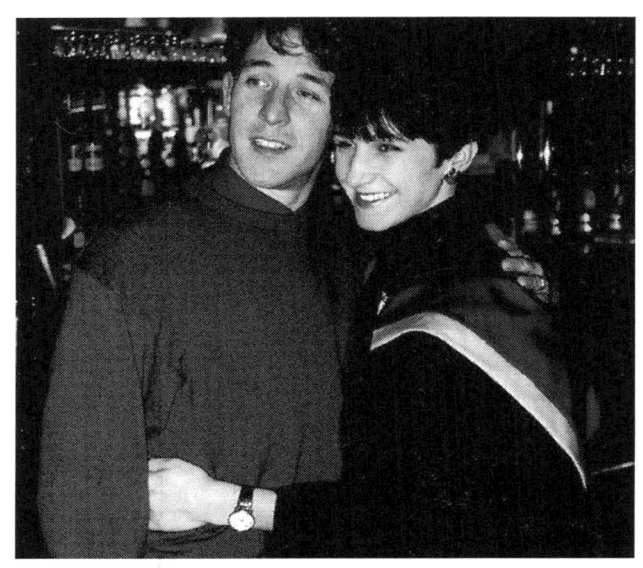

Mark and I at my graduation in 1992

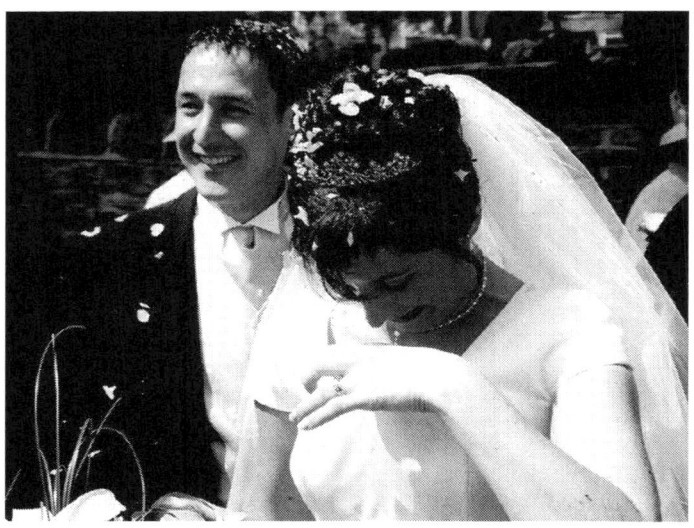

Mark and I on our wedding day in 1998

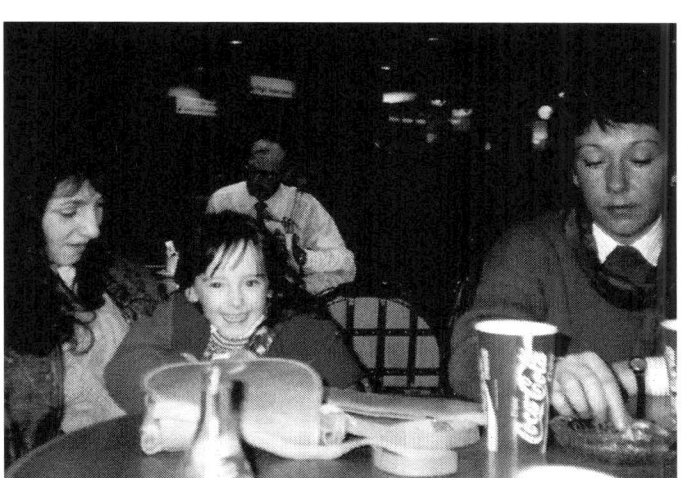

Saying goodbye to my mum and little sister Abi at Heathrow
Airport as I headed to America to start my new job as a nanny in
January 1989

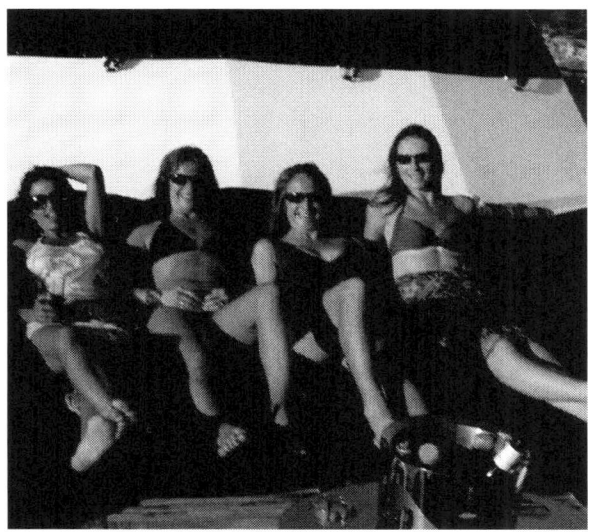

Joining the jetset for a day, Anita, Jaqui, Alison and I were
treated like stars by the owners of this yacht

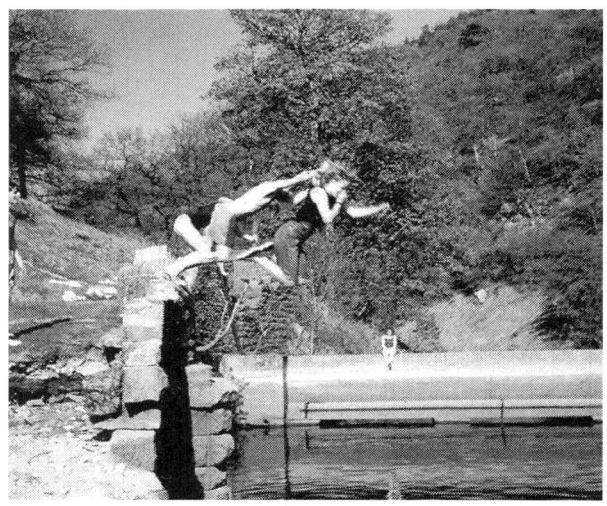

Mark and I diving into Derwent Reservoir summer 1991

Alison and I on holiday

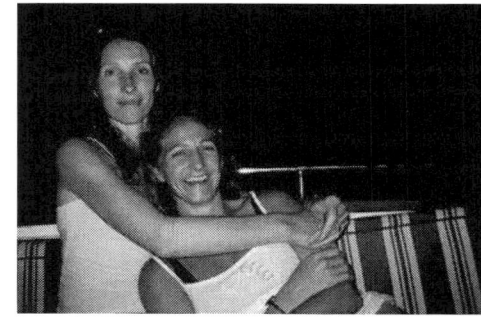

A family night out with my brothers, Paul and Tim, and my little sister, Abi

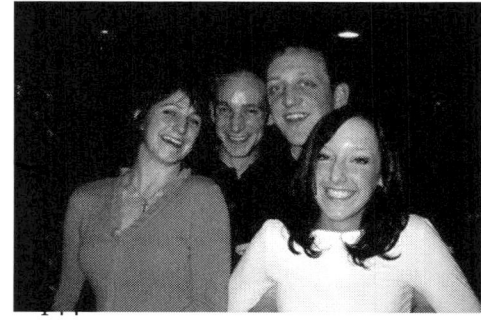

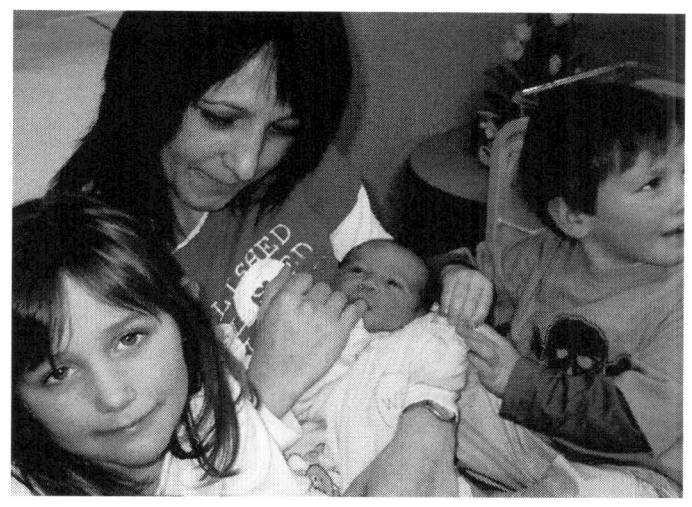

And then there were three. Harvey and India say hello to their baby
brother Woody, February 2004

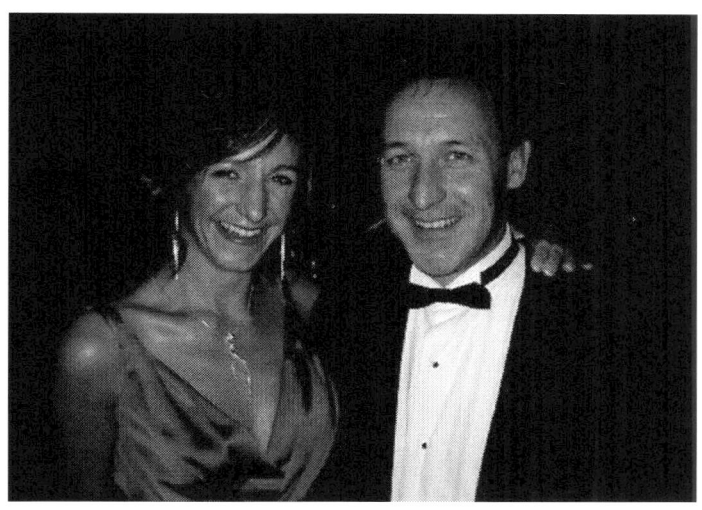

Mark and I having a ball

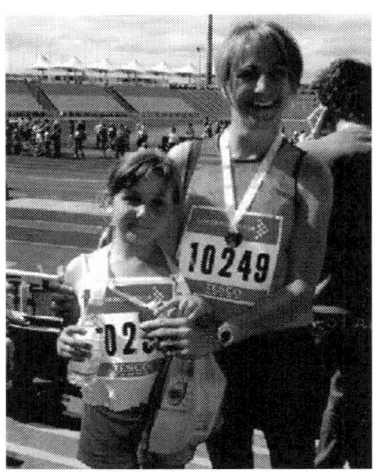

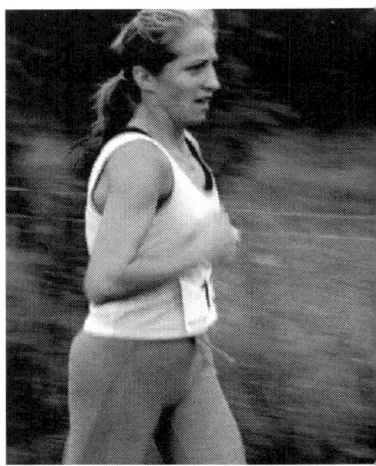

With my daughter, India,
at the finishing line of the
Sheffield Race For Life, 2006

Racing ahead, I completed the
Rother Valley 10k road race in
2007 in 42 minutes

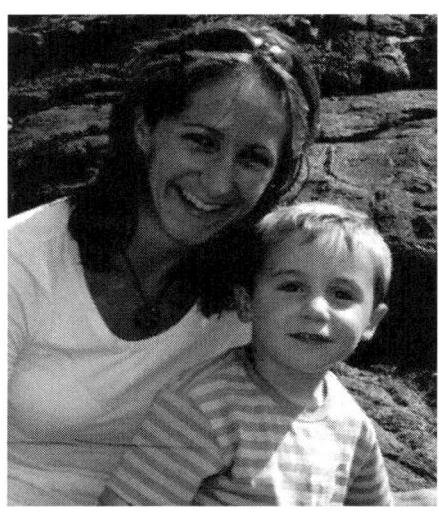

Woody and I on a family day out, summer 2008

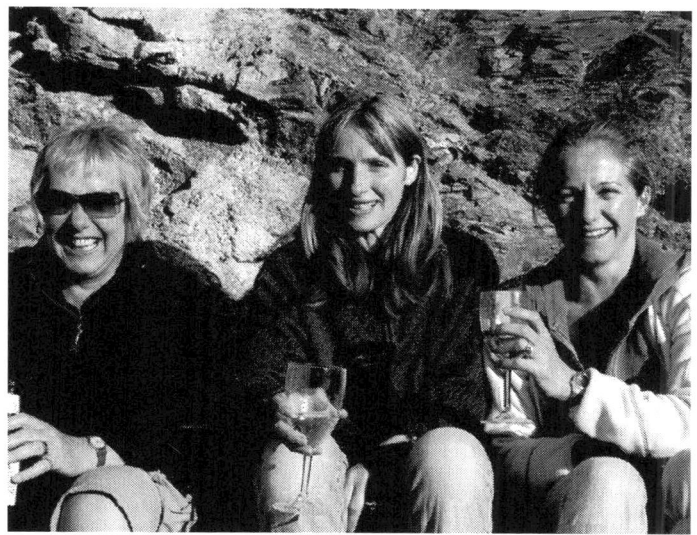
Mum, Alison and I enjoying a barbecue on the beach during our family holiday in Cornwall

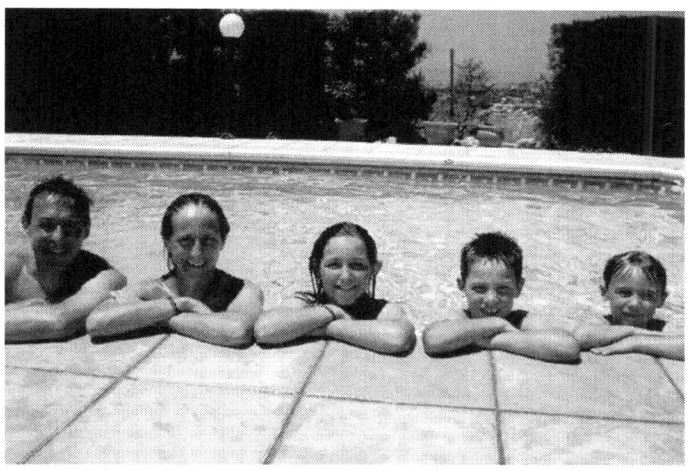
Water babies on holiday in Cyprus, 2009

147

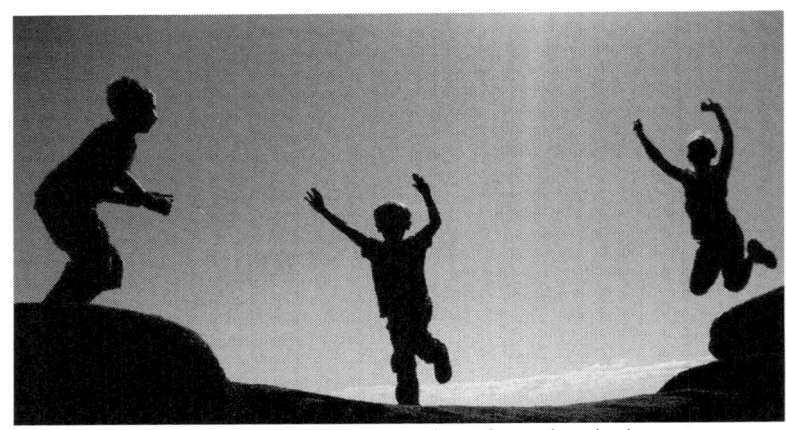

India, Woody, and Harvey at one of our favourite picnic spots, Burbage in the Park district

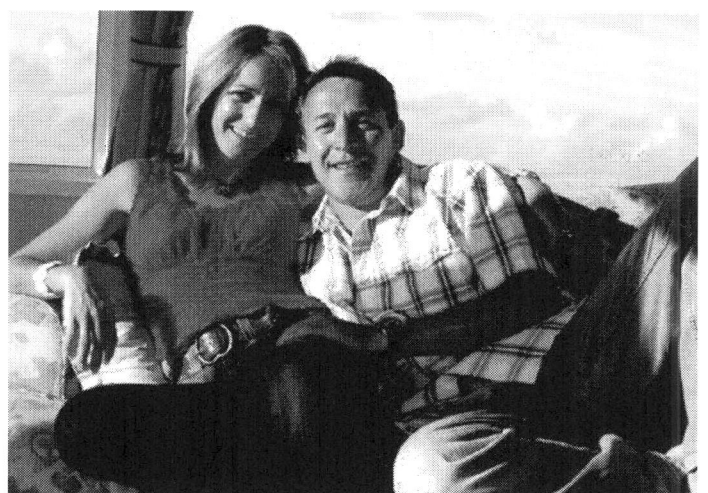

Mark and I relaxing

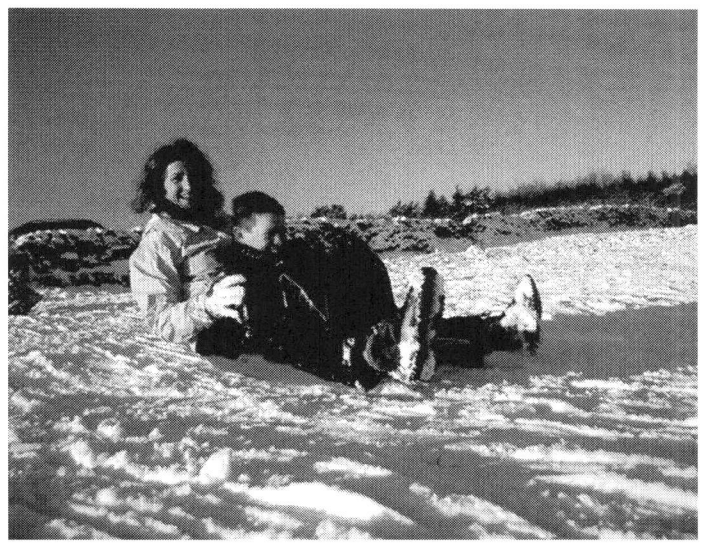

Big kids, Harvey and I sledging in the snow, winter 2009

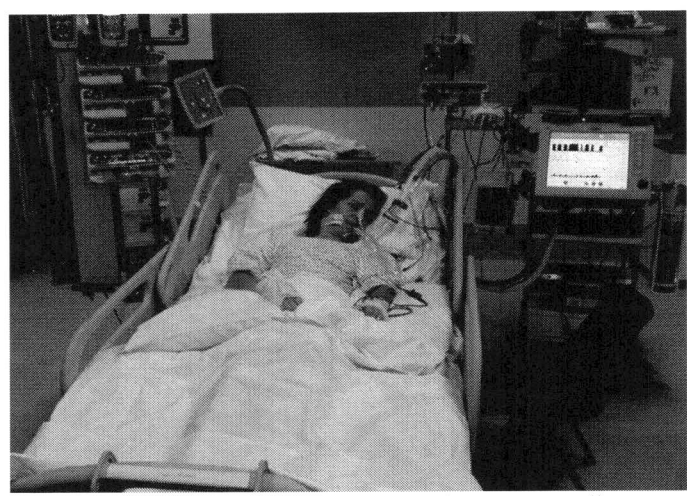

For three days after the stroke I was kept in a coma to allow my brain to recover. When I came round, I was locked in

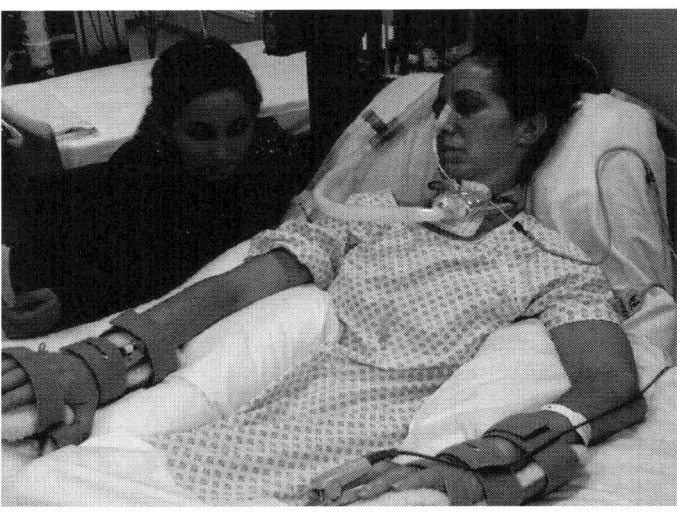

My daughter, India, was the first of our children to visit my in ICU, March 2010

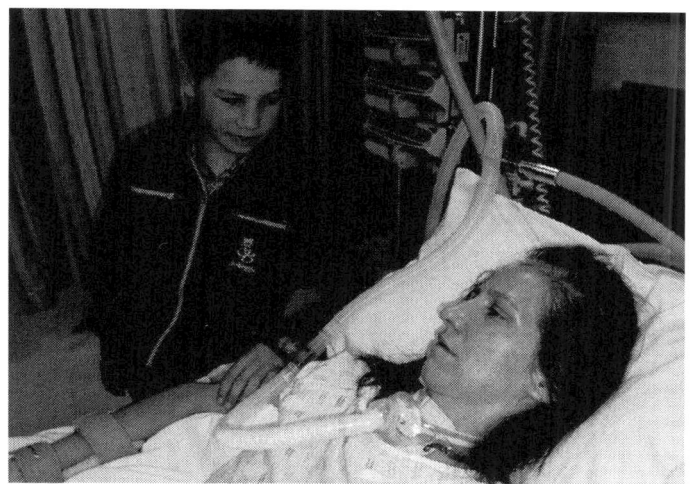

After he first saw me in hospital, Harvey went home and cried for two days

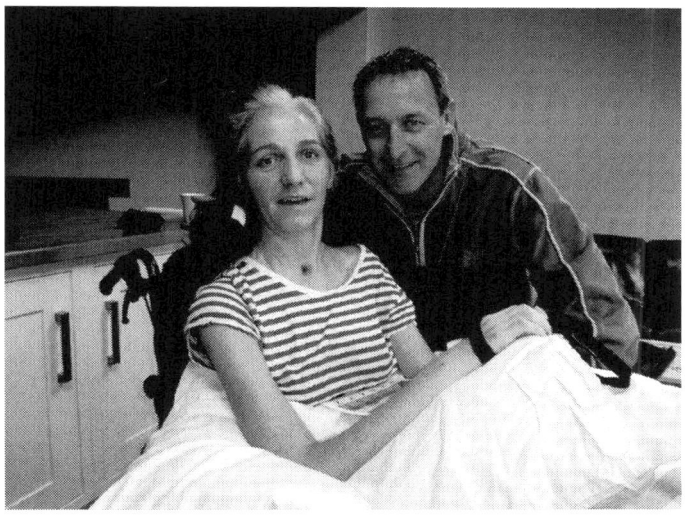

Mark and I during a day trip after I had my trachi out, leaving a scar on my neck

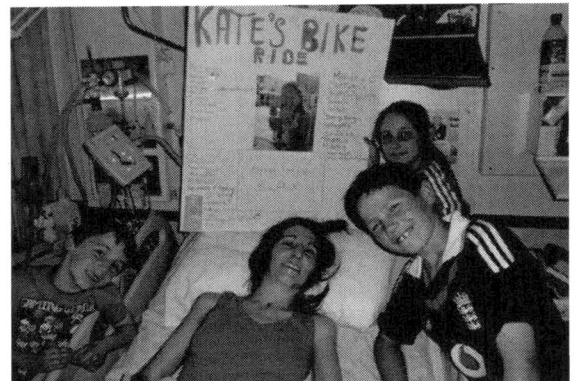

India, Harvey, and Woody were buzzing from their charity bike ride at Derwent Reservoir, May 2010

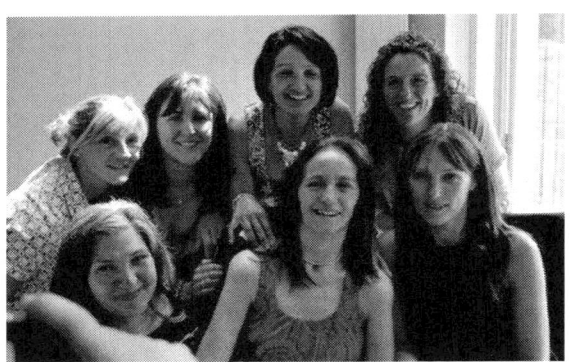

With my friends at my 40th birthday party

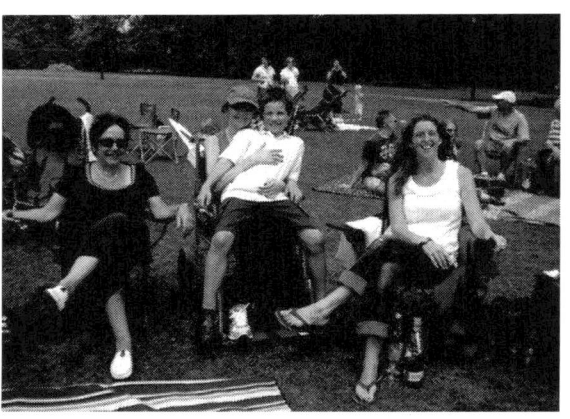

With Harvey and other school mums at Woody's sports day, June 2010

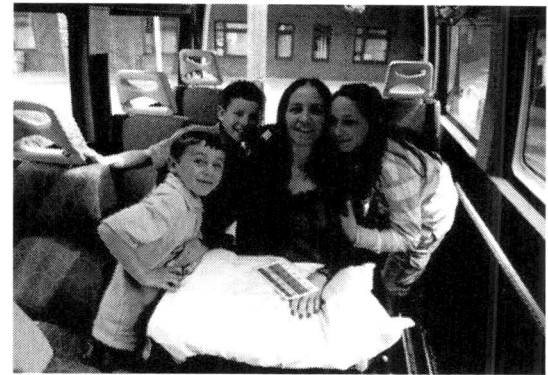

Day out in the hospital minibus with Woody, Harvey, and India, August 2010

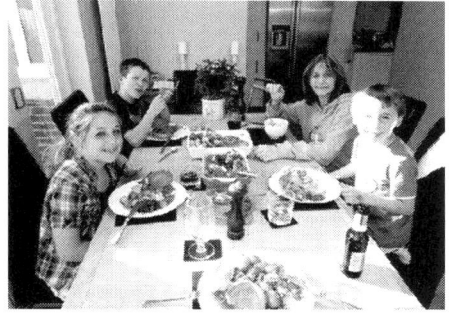

Home for the weekend I cooked my first roast dinner, September 2010

A	B	C	D	End of word
E	F	G	H	End of sentence
I	J	K	L	M	N
O	P	Q	R	S	T
U	V	W	X	Y	Z

The coloured letter chart became my way to communicate

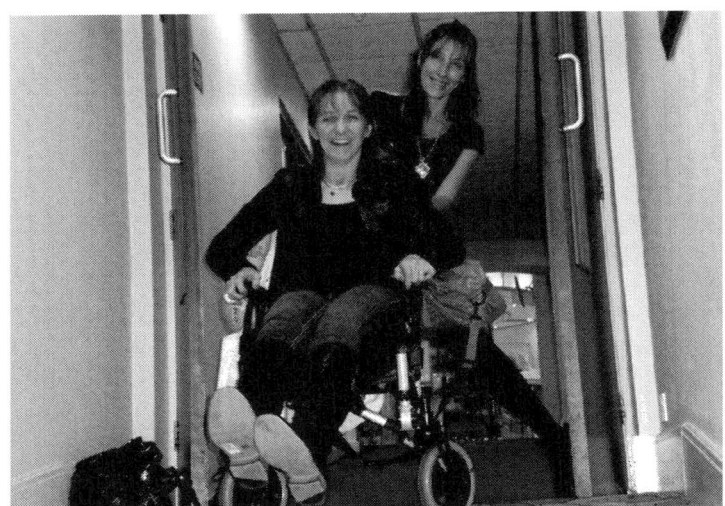

Driving Miss Daisy. Alison was my chaperone for a girlie weekend
away at Champneys Spa, October 2010

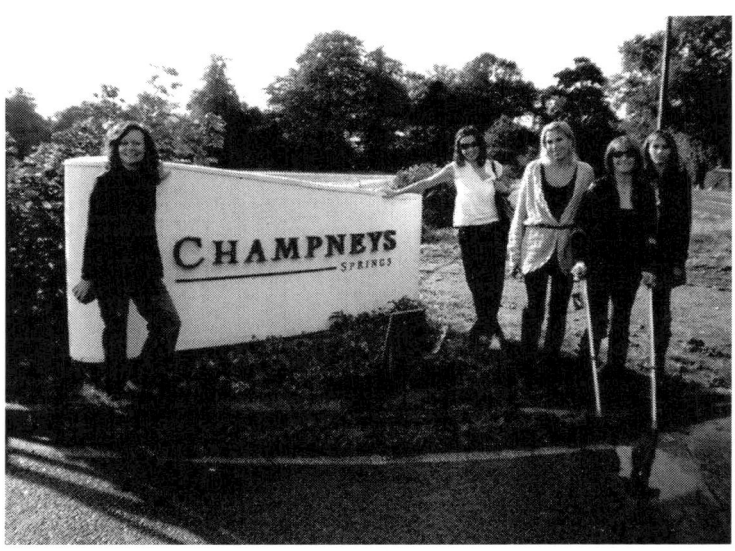

A spot of pampering on my first weekend away since leaving
hospital

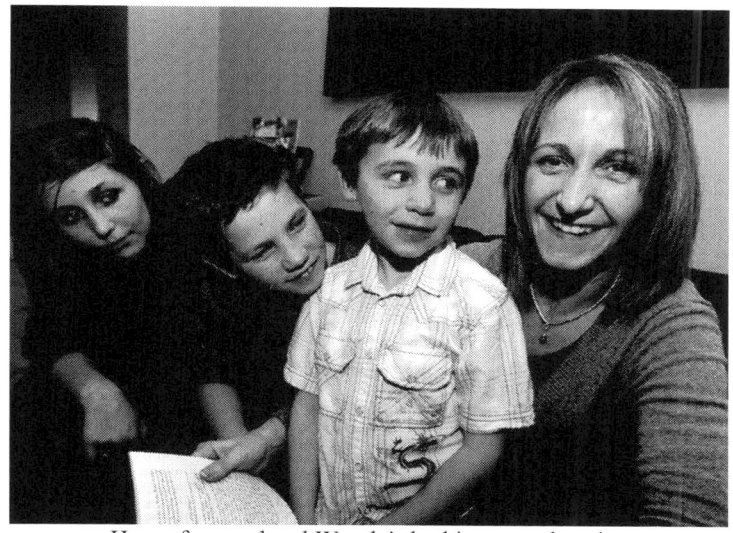
Home for good and Woody's looking apprehensive
©Star Newspapers

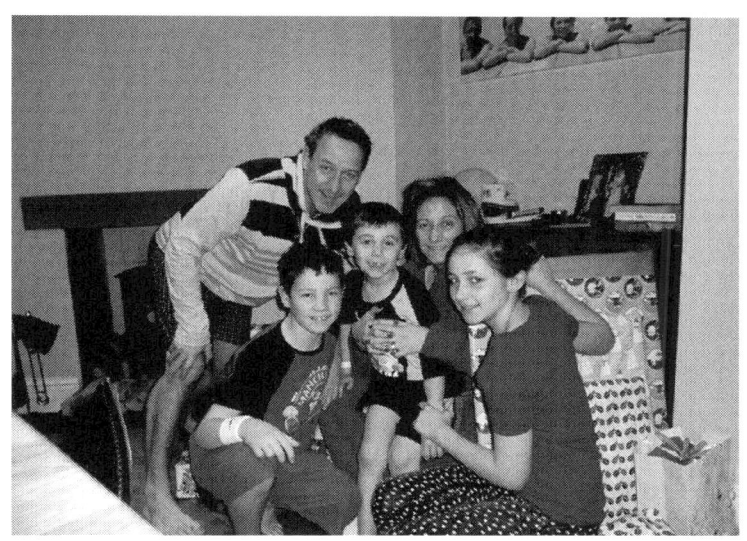
Christmas 2010 was special for my family

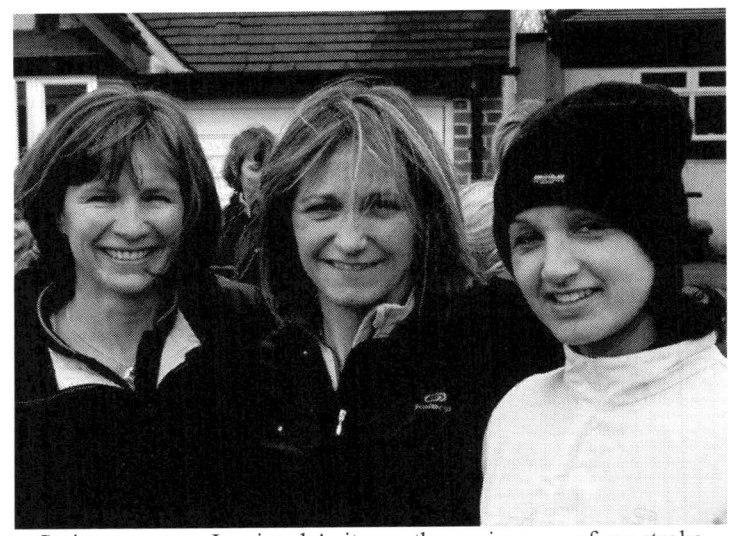

Serious runners, Jaqui and Anita, on the anniversary of my stroke

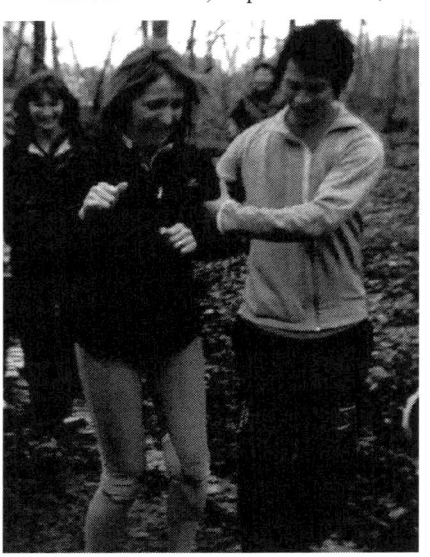

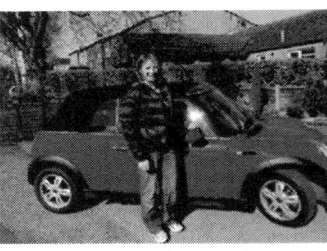

Freedom at last at the wheel of my new Mini convertible, nicknamed Rocky

My personal trainer Michael encouraged me to complete my first 20m run to mark the first anniversary of my stroke

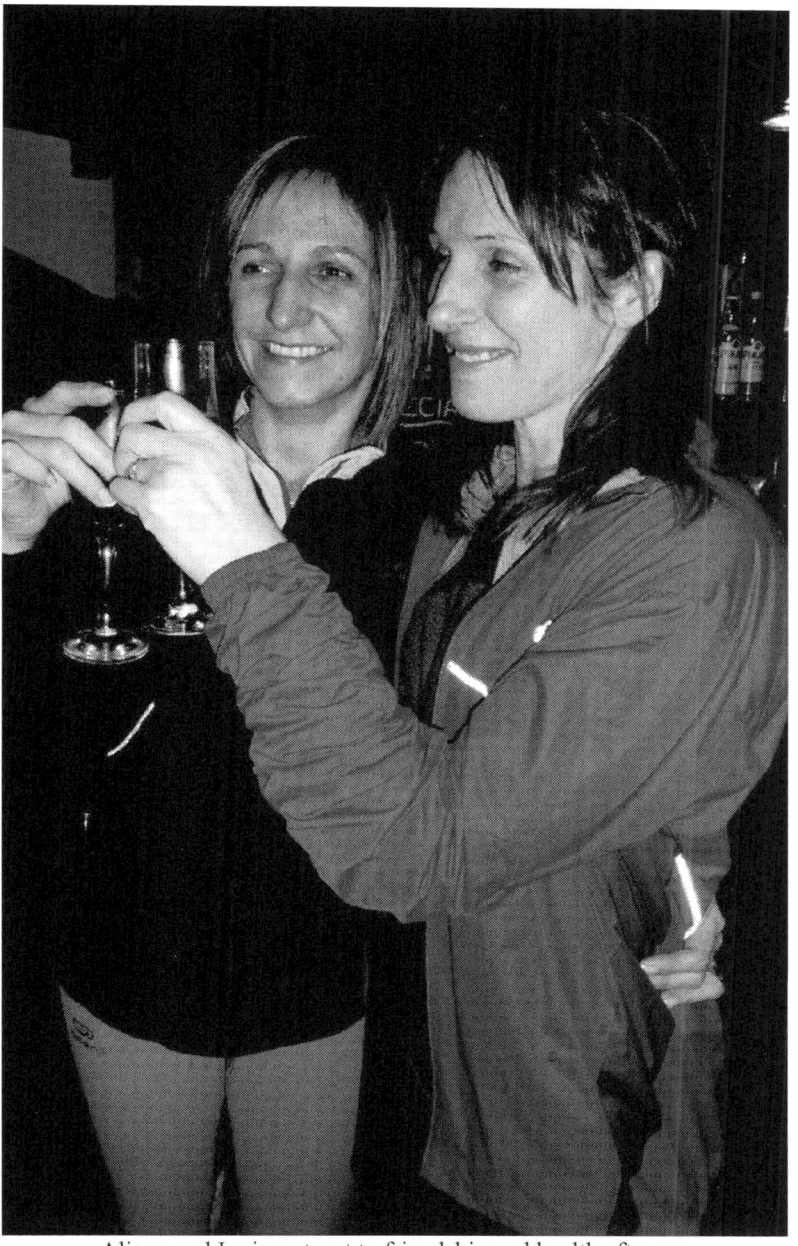

Alison and I raise a toast to friendship and health after my
anniversary fun run, February 6 2011

Chapter 26
Forty and not so Fabulous

NO WOMAN LIKES TO admit she's getting older, but for me my landmark fortieth birthday was more traumatic than I had anticipated. At the start of the year I had big plans to make my entrance into the fifth decade one to remember. It certainly was that, but not in the way I had planned. I could not even climb out of bed without two nurses and a hoist, so the ascent of Kilimanjaro was out of the question. As the big day, Thursday, June 3, approached, it also became clear that all the people I loved would be on holiday 330 miles away and I'd be stuck in hospital alone.

Every year around my birthday in June Mark, myself and the kids would join Alison and her family for a caravan holiday. Alison owned a caravan on a campsite near the coast of north Cornwall. I always liked to take the mickey out of her for being a middle-aged, middle-of-the-road 'caravanner', but it was actually one of those posh static caravans that some people like to refer to as a 'holiday home', and is more luxurious than some people's houses. Twice a year, in June and August, our family and another group of friends, the Manions, would rent caravans on the same site and we had some of the best times of our lives surfing, running up the sand dunes, swimming and cycling. Ever since Woody, and Alison's youngest child Nicole, who was just six months older and best friends with him, were babies we had always looked forward to our trips to Cornwall. Sometimes my mum and Dave brought their touring caravan to a nearby site and joined us. I remember once Mum babysat while Alison and I and our husbands went to dine at TV chef Rick Stein's seafood restaurant in Padstow. I don't remember much about the food, but I do recall having one of the best nights of the holiday. We laughed so much the people on the neighbouring tables thought we were roaring drunk, but we were just intoxicated by silliness and laughter.

This year was to be no exception. For my fortieth birthday we had planned a big barbecue on the beach, but as the departure day approached it became obvious that the party would be missing one person – the birthday girl. If you had asked me six months ago how I would like to spend my fortieth birthday, dribbling and wetting myself in hospital wouldn't have made the final list. But that was the reality. I could manage an afternoon trip off the ward but a week in a caravan the other end of the country was completely out of the question, in my therapist's opinion.

The news hit me hard. I had been pushing myself in therapy to make it happen. I was moving my right side, I was able to use a computer and I was making progress with my mouth exercises, but it wasn't enough. I was totally deflated. Mark being a bloke couldn't understand what all the fuss was about. After all it was only a birthday. But it was a big birthday. I could appreciate that Mark and the children needed a rest. Four months of juggling the day job, daily hospital visits and looking after the children was taking its toll on my husband. He was at breaking point. But as the departure day drew nearer I sank into a depression.

When Mark and the kids left on May 31, I was inconsolable. I felt like I had been abandoned by all the people I loved. My family and best friend were driving down to Cornwall, even Mum was away on a pre-planned trip of a lifetime across America and Canada for five weeks with one of her oldest friends. She had wrestled with her conscience over whether to cancel but felt she couldn't let down her friend. Fortunately my stepdad filled in the gap, lifting my spirits by reading a letter from Mum in which she talked about her and her friend sleeping in their car. 'I keep telling her they're not Thelma and Louise,' Dave laughed. Mum's letter ended with the words, 'My beautiful Kate with your wonderful, adoringly expressive eyes, I'm missing you terribly. Stay strong, be calm and BEHAVE.'

Behave? What could she mean? It wasn't as though I was a bad patient? Well, I was earning myself a reputation for being impatient and not listening but that was only because I had set myself a goal and was determined to go on holiday with my family. I wondered if this was the way the future would be. Life carrying on as normal for everyone except me.

Two days after Mark and the children had left, one of the nurses brought me a print-out of an email from Mark:

'Thought I would send you a little note, we have an email address for the Osborn 4 PC so they can let you read this and at least know what we are doing. Had an interesting start to the holiday. Packing. Got all kids stuff packed and also mine, so far so good. But nightmare, the roof pod does not fit the new car. Just what you need about six hours before you leave. Was left with no choice but trip to Halfords for new one. So got one and looks like I need to get the old one on eBay.'

Ha! Ha! I thought. It wouldn't have happened if I had been there to organise everything.

'Off we go, left at 3.10 a.m. It was a bit surreal with just the four of us. We have a new record. Two miles after we got on the motorway India was sick. Good job you told me about the sick bags and damage was not too bad. She couldn't even blame travelling in the back seat because she was in your seat up front!'

It was little comfort knowing that India had already taken my place in the role of mother. The email continued as Mark chronicled their weekend from boogie boarding on the beach, family dinners in the caravan, runs along the coastal path and days out in the drizzle. What he didn't mention was that when they arrived he hid himself away in the bedroom and cried uncontrollably. The email ended with:

We are thinking about you snuggle bum non stop. It's hard without you. Love you loads Kate
Mark XXXXXXX

Later I got one of the nurses to take me to the nurse's station and typed a reply:

I am so happy you are all having fun. I am typing this. My right hand is all working now as is right shoulder I will walk again. I am practising so hard. I am glad you are all having a break from caring for me. You both look tired. Anita is fab. She and Bill have found a park near hospital for Thursday. I am very excited for Indi's surf lessons. Dave was great yesterday when I had wobble. Have a fab holiday, but not too good without me. I am enjoying some freedom on keyboard. I love you and am enormously proud of you. Love Kate xxxxxx. PS keep typing.

The morning of my birthday another email arrived from Mark and the kids wishing me happy birthday with individual messages and lots of kisses from each of the

161

children. Anita had stepped in to save me from a totally miserable fortieth birthday by arranging to break me out of my hospital cell for just a couple of hours, which was all the nurses would allow. Although my trachi had been removed, I was still struggling to breathe and needed to have my cough reflex stimulated and be ventilated with an oxygen mask at fairly regular intervals. However Anita was not put off and after numerous meetings with my therapists and specialists it was agreed that I could manage a maximum of three hours out in my wheelchair before my bum would get numb. I drew up a guest list including my sister Abi, Mark's sister Jo, some of my old school friends and various mums from school and their children as it was the half-term school holiday. The venue chosen was Rivelin Valley Country Park as it was close to the Northern General Hospital and we would not waste too much time travelling. An ambulance was booked and on this occasion it was agreed I could go out without a nurse. However, before we were allowed out, Anita was appointed as my escort and given a crash course in nursing care should any disasters happen. She was shown how to use the emergency ventilator if my breathing took a turn for the worse. Fortunately I was OK, but one lady in the café needed resuscitating when Dave appeared wearing a nothing except a bright green mankini. It was Alison's idea of a long-distance joke. Before she left for Cornwall she had been out shopping and had packed a game of pass the parcel. Under every layer was a silly item of clothing with an instruction. There was a Nora Batty-style pinafore dress for me with the instruction, 'Wear this. I want a picture.' For Anita there was a plastic rain hat with more demands for photographic evidence. When it came to Dave's present – the green mankini made fashionable by Borat – there was a note stating, 'I do not want a picture'. But she got one. Dave being the great sport he is, sneaked off to the men's loo and swapped his chinos and short-sleeved shirt for his new beachwear and proceeded to parade around the park frightening small children and those of a nervous disposition. Not a good look for anyone – particularly a fifty-five-year-old, balding businessman. My friends roared with laughter and I even managed a lopsided grin. Abi managed to snatch a photo on her phone and sent it to Alison who was having a barbecue on the beach when the photo arrived. I'm sure I heard her shriek all the way from Cornwall.

Among all the laughter, the sadness hit me. I was drained physically and emotionally. Something as simple as a trip to the park had taken all the effort I had. Anita rounded the day off with a big white-iced birthday cake with forty candles. It looked real but was made out of foam and covered in icing. She had decided that if I couldn't eat it then neither could anyone else. It was a lovely gesture and as I feebly tried to blow out the candles with the help of my friends I made a wish … by my next birthday I would be back to normal.

After less than three hours, the ambulance minibus arrived and Anita loaded me into the back for our journey back to Osborn 4. As I looked through the window, all the smiling faces of my friends faded into the distance and I broke my heart. I cried so much that poor Anita ran out of tissues and had to resort to a pillow to mop up my tears. That made us laugh and then we started crying all over again.

Arriving back at hospital I was unceremoniously offloaded out of the ambulance and hoisted back into bed. Then the phone that Mark had given me before they left for Cornwall in order to stay in touch lit up with India's number. With my limited movement I was able to press the answer button and put the call on speaker-phone. I could hear the seagulls in the background competing with the massed family voices singing happy birthday to me. Just hearing India's voice gave me a lift. She passed the phone to Harvey, Woody and Mark and in turn they all talked of surf lessons and kite-flying, beach barbecues and boules. They all said they missed me, but they seemed to be having fun without me. After they hung up I felt a real emptiness.

Mark and the kids were looking tanned and refreshed when they returned home a day earlier than expected. They had decided to pack up and come home early and I can't say I was sorry. The children were buzzing with energy and excitement from their holiday and Mark was looking more relaxed than I remembered seeing him for ages. I was happy they had had such a good time in Cornwall but I was even happier to see them back home safely.

My birthday party away from my family created further problems for India, who was torn between going on holiday and staying by her mum's bedside. Although she was looking forward to surf lessons and swimming, she had wanted to be with me on my birthday. Alison had investigated the possibility of booking flights back from Cornwall for the two of them for the day, but there were no flights available and the six-hour drive was out of the question. To make matters worse some of her school friends were with their mums at the Rivelin Park party and this led to further jealousy and resentment. In India's mind they were traitors and for a while afterwards she could not bring herself to talk to them.

My next big event to look forward to was my visit home for my second birthday party, but beyond that I was thinking ahead to August and our next family holiday. I was determined that I would be back in the passenger seat for that one and joining the beach barbecues. I had missed my first and last family holiday. I set myself a new goal. By August I'd be well enough to join Mark and the children in Cornwall. I mentally made a note in my head that by August 21 2010 I would be a free woman, and started counting down the days.

Chapter 27
It's my Party and I'll Cry if I Want To

WHILE THE CARAVAN HOLIDAY had been a non-starter, there was never any question that I wouldn't be able to attend my own 'official' birthday party. It was part of my action plan and my therapy team had been helping me to prepare.

Several weeks before the date we had borrowed a wheelchair and my physiotherapist and occupational therapist (OT) had taken me home in the back of the hospital minibus so they could assess what was needed for my big day out. As I sat in the wheelchair waiting to be pushed over the threshold of my own home, it hit me just how far I still had to go if I was ever to return to a normal life. I thought back to the nights when I had staggered up the path, rather the worse for wear after a curry night out with the girls, and fumbled in my handbag for my front door keys trying not to make too much fuss and wake the children. Now the whole action of being led up the garden path took enormous effort.

The passage from the bus up our drive to the front door was straightforward, but the eight-inch-high step into our porch proved to be the barrier. The OT had borrowed a set of portable ramps from the hospital and, with a bit of muscle power, he was able to push me over the step and into the porch. It was a tight squeeze, but we made it.

Sunday June 6 arrived but I hardly felt like a party, which was out of character for me. Book Club, running sessions, visits to the hairdresser, I always managed to make them fun. That was me. But this party was being organised without me and I was really in no mood for it. I was also still recovering from my near-death brush with pneumonia and was feeling quite fragile and vulnerable. Alison had touched up my roots, so I knew that at least my hair was shining, even if the rest of me was limp.

When the nurses came to dress me that morning I had a new outfit to wear, which I had chosen with the help of Jo and a Next catalogue. Jo would often bring a catalogue on to the ward and allow me to choose pyjamas and clothes. She would hold the page in front of me, I'd blink once for no, she'd turn the page again until I eventually found something I liked. Then she would point to each photo on the page until I blinked on the one I liked. She would read out the colour choice and size, go home and place the order. Before I was able to go out shopping to Meadowhall, this method of shopping gave me a sense of purpose and control over how I looked. For my party I had chosen a bright green and pink, tunic-style top with short sleeves and a pair of jeans. I had lost so much weight, two and a half stone, that I had dropped two dress sizes and even a size six was hanging off me.

As the ambulance pulled into our street in Dore, I felt like the Queen, or even Katie Price. More than fifty people were waiting outside the house and in the garden; there was a big birthday banner hanging up in the front window and hundreds of balloons filled every space. I could tell that Alison, Anita, Jaqui and the children had been busy with the helium and paints. As the bus came to a halt children crowded around eager to look at the woman who cheated death. They wanted to hold my hand. It was suffocating, like being buried with kindness. I felt like a freak. But more than anything I felt totally dependent on others.

Mark wheeled me into the house using the ramps they had bought with my bike-run money. Inside, all my friends and family were waiting to greet me on this big occasion. Suddenly I was faced with a wall of memories. The last time Mark and I had been together in this house, he was panicking and I was being wheeled out on a stretcher. Now everything was reminding me of that fateful Sunday night. It was exactly four months to the day, something that had not crossed my mind until I was actually there. Hearing the children's footsteps on the stairs, seeing the rug where I had almost died in front of the television, were sudden reminders of my mortality. And now being home, with no crash team or ventilators on hand, scared me.

There was a false air of jolliness to the party; everyone seemed to be trying too hard to be happy for me. In addition to all my close friends, who had been by my bedside throughout the long journey, there were people there who had only known me as the fit young mum who ran through Dore. There were children from the school who only knew me as India, Harvey and Woody's mad mum who always won on sports day. What they were seeing was a different person from the one they remembered and I could sense it in the way they greeted me. It was all overwhelming. I tried my best to put on my crooked smile, but it was all a façade.

I was genuinely pleased to see my dad and his wife, Babs, who had made the ninety-mile journey from the

Wirral. He had been suffering from his own health problems. While I was in the ICU he had been diagnosed with a tumour in his bladder and had undergone his own treatment to have it removed. The last time I had seen him was when I was in the ICU and he had given me a teddy bear, to guard over me and show I was still his little girl. For two months after the operation he had been unable to travel long distance which meant that hospital visits were out of the question. Dad looked well considering he had been through surgery.

Once I had got over the initial shock of seeing so many people and being the focus of attention, it was time for the presents. India, Harvey and Woody took great delight in helping me to unwrap the gifts. There was the expensive watch I had chosen from Mark's parents, a bracelet from Tiffany and Co, New York from Alison, Anita and Jaqui, a silver bracelet from my mum and a selection of expensive moisturisers from the various Dore mums. The children showed me a Links of London jewellery box. 'This is from all of us and Daddy,' India, said proudly as she took out a beautiful silver heart-shaped pendant and hung it around my scrawny neck.

Last, but not least, Mark placed a glittering, silver rectangular box on my lap. It was about 18 inches long and tied up in a pink bow, which I guessed India had helped to decorate. I could guess what it might be. As Woody tore off the paper, I saw it was a netbook computer with my own dongle, which I could use to access the internet from my hospital bed. It was the gift I had been hoping for. The Grid 2 communication software which the staff at Osborn 4 had borrowed from another unit, had been useful as it had allowed me to access a computer screen using a switch, and in this way

169

I had managed to build up communication. But once I started using the PC on the nurses' station I had longed for a computer of my own. Using the Grid 2 I spelt out to Mark 'WANT A NETBOOK' And here it was.

Out of the corner of my eye I noticed Anita's expression drop. She had been in charge of placing the order for the Grid 2 software using £6,000 from the bike ride funds.

'What on earth are we going to do with the blooming thing,' when it arrives? We can't cancel the order. We've just wasted £6,000,' she whispered to Alison. Fortunately when it did arrive the hospital management bought it for use on Osborn 4.

After the present unwrapping, friends gathered in the kitchen, the place where so many of our previous parties always ended, to toast the birthday girl. I could not join in as I was still unable to drink at this stage, but I listened as they all voiced words of encouragement on how much I had improved and how they were convinced I would be home one day. Mark thanked everyone for their support to all the family during the rough times. Then Jaqui's husband, James, who is a man of great dignity and gentleness and considered in his words, asked if he could say something.

He began by saying how brilliant it was that I was home and how all my friends coming together showed what friendship is about. Then he said something that brought the entire room to silence. 'I'm sure we've all thought that we hope it never happens to our family.'

For a second there was a stunned hush as every eye in the room looked first to me then to their own loved ones. It was a brave thing to say out loud and coming from anyone else it could have been offensive, but James's words struck a chord.

The party came to an abrupt end when the nurses

decided that two hours was long enough for me to be out. I was drained emotionally and physically and still had the upheaval of being ferried into the minibus, wheeled out the other end and hoisted back into bed before I could relax again. As my wheelchair was locked into position in the back of the bus, the tears started to roll and I was overtaken by darkness. My friends read my tears as sadness to be leaving the party and all the people I loved. But I was relieved to be returning to my safe house at Osborn 4. My sadness came from the knowledge that there was such a long way to go before I could ever feel happy and secure in my old home. As the bus chauffeured me away I managed to lift my arm and give a regal wave.

Chapter 28
Therapy's Gone Mad

I HAD NEVER CONSIDERED myself a pushy person. I was a mum with high standards, who wanted to give her children every opportunity they had to develop their talents from a young age, which is why I made sure India, Harvey and Woody followed their timetable of activities. I would describe myself as driven and focussed, someone who sees failure as a sign of weakness. On Osborn 4 I quickly learnt that if you don't push, nothing happens very quickly.

After the crushing disappointment of being left alone during the family holiday to Cornwall, I was determined that I would be well enough to join Mark and the children for the main summer holiday in August. I set myself a new goal. I had two months to build up my physical strength and mobility so that I could get out. Like a prisoner given a parole date, I pictured an imaginary calendar in my head and with each twenty-four hours that passed and every new exercise I completed, I would cross off another day.

As my mum kept telling me, once you start to learn new movements, new pathways open up in your brain and you will never lose that connection. Although my progress had been slow to start with, I was encouraged by each new flicker. There are hundreds of muscles in the body controlling our movement and I had to relearn every single one. Yet everyday I was getting stronger and learning something new, and once I was given a new exercise I would practise and practise until I could do it. Over the weeks my friends and family started to see giant leaps in my recovery. As Alison kept telling me, I had my spark back. I had regained my fighting spirit and I was using it for positive progress. My mum recalled how amazed she had been when she came to see me after her holiday in America. When she had left me I was still in the high-dependency ward next to the nurse's station and was barely moving, when I needed to be taken out in the wheelchair I was always strapped in place and my facial expressions were limited. When she next saw me I had been moved to the larger ward next to a window, so I could look out at the trees and birds. I was able to hold myself in an upright sitting position and I was able to smile, it was a gaping, toothy grin, but it showed I had regained some control of my facial muscles. The tongue-waggling and ping pong ball-blowing exercises were having an effect.

However I was still craving my Earl Grey tea and before they would allow me to start drinking again I had to pass a videofluoroscopy test, which would determine if I was capable of swallowing without choking. To prepare for the test, Sophie the speech therapist set me a programme of exercises to improve my ability to swallow. Sitting upright in my wheelchair, my helper would bring me a half-full beaker of ice and a teaspoon from the ward kitchen. The teaspoon would be put in my mouth, just as if they were feeding a baby, the coldness of the spoon was supposed to help trigger my swallow reflex. I could feel and taste its icy metalness on my tongue as it pressed down. The spoon was completely dry to avoid any unwanted moisture trickling into my lungs but sometimes I imagined it contained a mouthful of my favourite roast chicken dinner and clamped my mouth shut. The object of this exercise was to get me to close my lips around the spoon allowing the person holding the spoon to pull it out. Sometimes the therapy team conducted the exercise but Mark, Alison and Anita also learnt the drill and would practise with me during the visiting hours. Initially it was pretty hit and miss, the action of having a foreign object in my mouth would make me clamp my mouth shut like a dog with a bone and my helper would have to gently prise the spoon out of my grip. But within the space of a couple of days I had become accustomed to this invasion of cutlery; I got more experienced at closing my lips only around the spoon and swallowing the saliva which my mouth produced.

As the movement in my right side grew stronger I was able to practise a more advanced version of this exercise, where I was allowed to feed myself with actual water while sitting up in my wheelchair. Again it started feebly, with a lot of spluttering and missing of the mouth until I was allowed a whole ten half-teaspoons of cold water five times a day.

When the time came for my first videofluoroscopy I was wheeled down to the X-ray unit and given a thick barium mixture to drink. I was parked in front of the camera and waited as the machine moved up and down in front of my neck photographing my oesophagus as the mixture slid down into my stomach. After it was all over my speech therapist came back with my results. I had failed as the muscles in my food pipe were too weak; they weren't doing the job of pushing the food down. I was absolutely gutted as had it never crossed my mind that I wouldn't pass the test. I had to wait another month before I could try again.

While this was a blow, I was kept positive by my physiotherapy which was improving in leaps and bounds. My physio had drawn up a list of exercises, which were taped to the side of my locker...

Kate's Exercises

1. In lying or sitting position; hold upper arm and wrist and slowly lift arm up and down. Kate will guide on how far to go. She needs more help with the left arm. Repeat 10 times and then take the arm out to the side.

2. In sitting position, put chair in upright position and assist Kate into a more forward position from her lower back. Keeping your hand on her lower back, encourage Kate to 'slump, then sit up' without overusing her head.

3. When sitting unsupported forwards in chair; practise lifting right hand up.

4. Lying with knees bent and feet flat on the bed, assist Kate to hold her knees and feet steady while she does 10 SLOW bottom lifts and lowers.

These movements were aimed at strengthening my slack muscles to help me regain my balance, which would determine whether I was strong enough to attempt walking. When Mark, Mum, Alison or Anita visited I would stare at the exercise chart and they'd go through the routines with me while chatting. They gave me a sense of purpose and I'm sure they helped me achieve my goals much quicker than my therapists had expected.

With two nurses and a hoist I was managing to stay upright for longer, which meant I could start working towards getting on and off the toilet and in time I could get rid of the catheter bag. I was learning how to push myself up into a standing position from the wheelchair.

I was even becoming more comfortable sitting in a wheelchair all day, which gave me greater freedom to move around the ward and spend time at the nurse's station, where I could use Facebook.

On June 24 I proudly announced via Facebook:

I walked today with some help.'

Leading up to this major achievement, my physiotherapist had introduced me to the walking frame. If the tilt table had been Frankenstein's bed, the walking frame was a giant baby-walker. It consisted of a sturdy metal frame on wheels with a thick leather belt in the centre and handles at the front. I was held into position and strapped tightly into place with the belt. Then Gemma, my physiotherapist, encouraged me to move my legs. At first I needed her help as she moved my right foot into a forward step, followed by my left. We did it again, right then left. Then she stood in front of me and I repeated, right then left. I was walking. It was not a pretty sight, but it was forward motion. I had the biggest grin on my face. In my head I was following a rhythm, 'fuck you, fuck you, fuck you,' I was saying to all those nay-sayers who told my family I would never walk again.

'Look, Kate is walking!' Gemma called across the ward to Oliver, who was checking one of the patients' catheter bags.

'Hey, you were right. You always told me you would walk again, now look at you go,' he replied, making me feel 10ft tall as I took one clumsy step after another. I heard a ripple of applause as the nursing staff and patients cheered me on to further strides.

After this I wanted more and more. I thought, if I can walk then I can run, but my physiotherapist was more cautious and tried to hold me back by taking it one step at a time.

It was also a significant step into a future where I would not be dependent on a wheelchair. One of the first books I read when I was able to move my hand was *'Don't Leave Me This Way Or When I Get Back On My Feet You'll Be Sorry*. It was written by Julia Fox Garrison, a young American mum who had also suffered a massive stroke and was told she would never walk again. I related to her both psychologically and physically. But I particularly empathised with her frustrations at being stuck in a wheelchair. For most people just seeing a wheelchair rightly or wrongly conjures up ideas of sickness and disability. It also brings out the patronising side in people, who just can't seem to stop themselves from talking down to you. Just because you are unable to use your legs, they also assume that you also cannot use your brain and you are probably deaf too, so they speak to you loudly and slowly, emphasising every syllable. This really annoyed me and I thought to myself – if people are going to treat me like an invalid them I'm going to exploit it as much as I can. This attitude came as something of an embarrassment to Alison who was the one who had to act as my mouthpiece when demanding special disabled dispensations. On one of our day trips to Meadowhall shopping centre I saw a dress that I thought India would like but she was in school. 'Ask the assistant to keep it for me,' I blinked to Alison, knowing that I would be going back to the shop a couple of days later with India. So Alison left me near the door, as it was too difficult to manoeuvre the wheelchair through the cramped racks of clothes, and went off to ask for the favour. Sorry, can't do. It's not store policy, came the reply.

'Tell her I'm in a wheelchair,' I insisted. At this point Alison was too embarrassed to go back. 'Tell her,' I demanded with one of my killer stares. As Alison went back to talk to the shop assistant, I waited. The assistant looked across to me and I adopted the most pitiful expression my slack facial muscles could manage. It worked. Result. 1-0 to the lady in the invalid chariot. Another time Alison was convinced we'd get lynched when I forced her to push me to the front of the queue in Primark. No one dared complain, it just wouldn't have been PC. In time my friends nicknamed me 'Andy' after the comedy character in the TV series *Little Britain* who runs off and does able-bodied things while his carer's back is turned. This made me laugh as it was just the sort of thing I would do and now I was learning to walk again, I was thinking I might just do it.

*   *   *

Through using the computer mouse and keyboard to log on to my Facebook account the co-ordination was returning to my right hand. My fingers were able to grip the mouse and move it around the desk, and with a bit of effort I could exert just enough pressure to click it. I was also able to separate the fingers on my right hand enough to hit the keys on the keyboard. The freedom it gave me to write messages was a great boost to my mental health. The communication board had its uses, but I was impatient. Waiting to spell out every letter was time-wasting: with a computer screen I could voice my achievements quickly.

A couple of days after my first steps I wrote on Facebook:

I have progressed to a walking frame. Later I was so tired I passed out. Shh don't tell physio.

As I pushed ahead with therapy, I became conscious of hiding my exhaustion from the nurses and therapy team. Walking just a few steps was even more tiring than running a marathon. The therapists had their rules to follow, evolved from years of research and

178

experience with other head-injury patients, I had a mission to get better and go home. I was afraid if I ever showed I was tired or too weak they would reduce my therapy and there was no way I was going to let that happen.

A month later the exercise chart on my locker was replaced with a new one. My therapists often said that as soon as they drew up one action plan, I moved the goal posts. It often felt like I was pushing them, rather than the other way round.

The new exercises involved lying on my bed with a wedge under my legs. I had to pull my toes towards my body, slowly straighten my knee then lower my foot back to the wedge. I had to do this five times then swap legs, aiming for three sets on each leg. With the help of another person I also had to stand with a walking frame in front of me to balance myself then unlock my knees and let go of the frame. If I found this too easy I had to add some slow head turns and hand raises.

Another exercise was standing with my fingertips on the walking frame, I had to bend my knees and straighten up again. I had to repeat this in sets of five, three sets at a time. My therapist warned me that if I started to shake or wobble I should stop, and when I was with them I had to. But when I was on my own or with my family I would keep pushing until I shook with exhaustion. Again these were all exercises designed to improve my muscle strength and stamina. When faced with any new set of exercises I employed my running psyche based on the importance of setting objectives beyond my ability. I thought back to the previous summer when I had signed up to run the Sheffield half marathon, the first major long-distance event I had entered. My aim was to complete the 13.1 mile course in one hour and forty minutes, a good ten minutes faster

179

than any of my previous best times. Mark scoffed, but on the day I pushed myself harder and finished in one hour thirty-eight minutes. Setting hard and demanding objectives was in my blood and therapy was no exception.

By August I started learning to dress myself again, another long and laborious task. I had been wearing lots of loose clothes, tracksuit trousers with elasticated waists and baggy T-shirts which were all unflattering but didn't obstruct my PEG. With the help of a nurse it took me more than an hour to get dressed. Getting my top on was a palaver as I could not control my movement enough to lift my T-shirt over my head. Pulling on my trousers was also hard work as I did not have the balance to stand up and step into them, nor did I have the flexibility to sit on the edge of the bed and pull them over my feet, so this required some help. But tying my shoelaces was the most difficult task. My fingers were so undexterous that each time I tried to make a loop with the lace, it would undo. Five hours it took me to tie my first shoelace. I remember sitting next to Oliver at the nurses' station hour after hour with my trainer on my lap, fumbling with my laces and cursing under my breath. But like everything else, I would not give up till I'd tied the damned thing.

Chapter 29
Wheelbarrows and Friendship

I LOVED BEING OUTSIDE in the hospital garden, as I have said before. It gave me a sense of freedom and the fresh air was a welcome change from the stuffiness of the ward. When I was poorly I always had to be well-wrapped in a fleecy blanket, but the sensation of the breeze on my face reminded me of being outdoors and running. I would have been happy to have my bed wheeled out there permanently.

The garden outside Osborn 4 was nothing special. There was a patio leading on to a patchy area of grass where a lawn had once been. There were a couple of plastic chairs dotted around, a garden bench and a raised flower bed which had long been neglected and resembled a jungle. The grass sloped down to a row of trees and beyond that the road, which for me symbolised freedom. From my wheelchair viewpoint I could look across the valleys and see the villages of north Sheffield in the distance. This was another of my favourite running routes. Many a weekend Anita and I would run through fields of Highland cattle with their enormous horns. I was reminded of a time when we had taken Anita's Dalmatian dog, Cai, out running with us. While the dog was sniffing for rabbits in the field, the cattle started to charge towards us. You've never seen Anita and I run so fast; we grabbed the dog and leapt the fence to safety.

Inside the ward as I was gaining mobility I was also making new acquaintances with the other long-term patients. Mavis was another one who loved being outdoors. She was an active woman of sixty, who ran a bowling team and was something of a sun-worshipper until she contracted encephalitis from a cold sore and ended up severely disabled. In the summer months she would join me in the garden where she sat on the grass and soaked up the sun. After I returned home I learnt that she too left hospital and now lives in a nursing home nearby, as it was decided she could never look after herself again.

In the bed next to mine lay a Muslim woman from Somalia. I never really found out what was wrong with her as she was intensely private and spoke very little English. She never socialised with the other patients at meal times and I only ever saw her black/brown eyes through the tiny slit in her burkah, which she wore at all times. She spent a lot of time praying behind the curtains which she would often draw around her bed when her visitors arrived to block out the rest of the ward. I sensed that she was even more of a pain to the nurses than I was. She didn't allow the nurses to help her in the shower, which was a worry for them as they were afraid she could fall and hurt herself. She did, unintentionally, make me laugh one afternoon when Alison was visiting. I can't remember what the two of us were talking about but we were laughing, probably quite loudly. Unnoticed by us the Somalian woman got out of bed and crossed over to my bay, looked at Alison and said 'You poorly'. To which Alison replied that she was not a patient, she was just visiting. 'No, you poorly,' the woman in the burkah insisted and turned back to her bed leaving Alison and me puzzled and struggling to stifle our laughter. I can only assume that she heard Alison's raucous laugh and thought she was struggling to breathe.

Another of my ward friends was a young Asian boy who had suffered a massive brain injury in a car accident and was left permanently in a wheelchair. He was something of a boy racer and when I was promoted to the use of an electric wheelchair which I could control on my own, he often challenged me to races along the ward, which got us into trouble with the nurses but was great fun. I later discovered that he had crashed his car on the dual carriageway when he was hanging out of the window and showing off. This knowledge changed my feelings towards him. It also made me feel more self-pity. From that point I could not look at him without thinking, you are in that wheelchair because of your own stupid fault. I had no choice.

I was sitting out in the garden with Mavis and the burkah lady one hot sunny afternoon when I saw Anita's white Mercedes van pull up in the car park. To my surprise Anita and Alison got out each carrying a spade and a garden fork. I had no idea what they might be up to and they were not due to visit according to my visitor's timetable for the day. Anita started to unload a wheelbarrow full of plants out of the back of the van. When she noticed me in the garden she waved and carried on regardless. What followed was like watching an episode of *Ground Force,* without Alan Titchmarsh. Anita had been to the local garden centre in Dore and explained about my stroke and the uninspiring jungle of a garden that was all the patients had to look at. The owner had agreed to let her buy a load of plants at cost price and the ward manager gave her permission to make over the plot. All this was done without a word

183

being mentioned to me, it was meant to be a surprise. It was another of those thoughtful gifts that showed her caring nature. Between the two of them Alison and Anita spent the afternoon transforming the flower bed into something worthy of Kew Gardens.

As I watched them work I realised again how lucky I was to have such good friends. Anita, Jaqui and Alison were three very different characters but each was strong and independent. Anita was the caring one with a heart-of-gold, Jaqui the practical and knowledgeable one and Alison, as I have said many times before, was my soul-mate. I thought how my illness had brought these women closer together. There was a time when it would be fair to say that Anita treated Alison with suspicion. For starters Alison had no interest in running, which was a black mark against her in Anita's books, and she had a naughty, almost child-like sense of fun, which Anita probably disapproved of as being a little bit immature. I remember Anita being shocked one day when Alison and I turned up to pick the children up from school covered in grazes and bruises. The night before we had been drinking after closing time at Alison's hair salon and after one glass of Shiraz too many, thought it would be fun to ride downhill on Alison's hairdressing stools. And it was fun ... until we collided in a heap at the bottom of the hill like a pair of reckless teenagers after a night on cheap cider. Gradually, as Anita and Alison started bonding at my bedside, she too came to know Alison's warm and friendly nature. Sometimes I watched them leaving together after a visit and feel a certain comfort in the fact they had 'found' each other as friends even if I was a bit jealous that I couldn't be with them.

Neither Alison nor Anita were green-fingered but that afternoon they turned that bit of ground into an area of outstanding natural beauty. It was a sea of vivid red, sunny yellow and beautiful blue flowers. As they worked I couldn't help but notice the male nurses were admiring another natural beauty. They could not take their eyes off Anita. She was wearing very skimpy white shorts and a tight white vest that showed off her curves in all the right places and with big pink gardening gloves to stop her hands getting dirty, she looked like a coffee-skinned Charlie Dimmock. I wasn't surprised that the men were mesmerised by her earthy curves. I felt a pang of jealousy as I wondered if I would ever look good in shorts again. It had been months since I last felt feminine and fanciable. In my current state I had become invisible to the opposite sex. Even Mark looked at me as if we had more of a brother/sister relationship, and kissed me with dry lips when all I wanted was to feel desired.

Chapter 30
Day Trips and Diaries

I WAS NOT ALWAYS the easiest of patients to care for, it has to be said. I have since discovered that it is not uncommon for some people to suffer personality changes following a severe stroke. In particular, active men, who were used to being the breadwinners, can become severely depressed by the loss of their mobility and ability to work. I could not say that this was the case with me. I had always been impulsive, determined and a straight-talker, hot-tempered if you were to ask Mark. When I was locked in I had no way of expressing myself. Initially some of the nurses had thought I was posh, until one of them caught me giving them the 'rods'.

The 'rods', as we say in Yorkshire, is a slang term for the two-fingered gesture that we all know. As my right arm grew stronger I found new ways to express my impatience. Mark, who was usually the person on the receiving end of my two-fingered hand signals, was used to it but the nurses were rather shocked that this fragile young mum from Dore could be so offensive. If things weren't happening quickly enough I would flip the rods. When I buzzed to be taken to the toilet and was told 'in a minute' I would give the nurse the rods. It made me feel better if nothing else, and it was exercising my right arm.

In spite of my bad behaviour, the nurses started allowing me out for a couple of hours at a time. The first test had been the shopping trips to Meadowhall and the visits home and to the park for my birthday party. Despite the emotional baggage that came with these trips, physically they were considered a success and I was allowed out more regularly. These days still involved quite a bit of organising. Before I could go anywhere either my family or the nurses had to arrange the wheelchair-adapted minibus. It was always in demand and usually needed to be booked at least a week ahead. I also required two nurses with me, so a trip out could never be made on the spur of the moment.

We started off with an afternoon at home at the weekend. It was only a two-hour release for me, but for Mark and the children it took up half of their day as they had to make the thirty-minute drive across town to the hospital to accompany me into the minibus for the drive back home. Then at the end of the afternoon they would have to do the same, unload me, settle me in and drive back home. I have to say that on these occasions the children were on their best behaviour, Mark had warned them.

Initially these trips were painful. I would sit in my wheelchair in the corner of our open plan kitchen/diner where I had spent so much time together with the children and feel my eyes welling up with tears. The smells and sounds of being home, the sound of Harvey opening the fridge door for a drink, the computer-generated noise of Woody and India playing on the Nintendo Wii in the playroom next door, even the happy smiling family portrait on the wall of the five of us all lined up and grinning in a swimming pool on holiday, reminded me of what I was missing.

The children would sit beside me and say, 'Come on, Mummy, be happy. You're home with us.' And I tried, but it wasn't easy. They would show me their school work, and pictures they had drawn for me during the week. India was the creative one and made pretty floral collages for me. Harvey would run out into the garden to show me his latest football trick and Woody just sat on the sofa as close to my chair as possible and held my hand, looking at me. In his huge expressive eyes, which he inherited from me, I could see he wanted his old, normal mummy home for good. Most afternoons we used the communication board but the children found it even more difficult to master than the adults. I would spell out things like 'HAVE YOU BEEN TO BEAVERS?' to Woody or 'DID YOUR TEAM WIN?' to Harvey.

One afternoon I was in the middle of spelling out a message to the children when Woody got bored and said, with the impatience of a six-year-old, 'Why don't you just write it?' handing me a pen and a notepad. How could I let him down? I took the pen in my shaky right hand while Woody held the pad for me. At first I could not put enough pressure on the page and the pen slipped, leaving inky lines across the paper. Then I tried again, concentrating on making my hand follow the letters I could so see clearly in my head. I had to do it before Woody lost interest. The W was easy, straight down and up. The Os and the D were more difficult as I needed to move my hand in a circular motion, which I had not practised. Then I added a Y. It was a shaky and childish attempt at writing. In the corner of my eye I could see Mark filling up with tears as he watched from the other side of the kitchen. He thought Woody had been cruel to make me do something that was beyond my capabilities, but he had just pushed me to reach another goal quicker than anyone had expected.

Having written Woody's name on paper, I couldn't leave India and Harvey out. They too wanted me to write their names. Slowly, concentrating hard on my hand and the pen, I scrawled their names too.

When I returned to hospital after this visit, the staff were once again amazed by my progress. Mark and the children left me with a notepad on my bed and all night I practised writing the names of all my friends and the people I knew, until I got so tired my handwriting degenerated into an illegible childish scribble. Writing gave me another new freedom to express myself. I would write down my demands to the nurses. When I was on my own in bed I was also able to record my thoughts and feelings. Writing was something I could do impulsively, as long as I had a notepad and pen left close to my hand. Left alone in my own thoughts, I started to write my thoughts down in a diary, which became the starting point for this book.

During the home visits I worried about what would happen if my catheter bag overflowed or my nappy needed changing. When I had nurses accompanying me I felt I was in safe hands but after a month or so of these visits I was allowed out without nurses and that's when my fears were magnified. Mark took over the responsibility as my prime carer. Although he had been by my side through the entire journey, he had never had any hands-on experience with my medical care, so he had to be given lessons in how to change my catheter bag. In hospital these things were taken for granted, when I had a full bag, the nurses would draw the curtains around my bed, switch off the tube to the bag, change it for an empty one, open the tube again, job done. At home the potential embarrassment of my bag overflowing and dripping onto the floor in front of my children became a worry which magnified in my head so much that I never felt I could relax and enjoy my time out and always felt a sense of relief when I went back to hospital.

In addition to the weekend visits home with Mark and the children, I was also allowed out during the week when Mum and Dave or Alison were at home to look after me. Anita would pop in for coffee and for a few minutes it felt like old times, except that I was unable to join in the chatter without the communication board. These days out were made easier once I learnt to stand on my own and could slide from the wheelchair into a normal car seat. That meant I did not have to rely on the minibus for day trips and could stay out as long as I liked. If I felt like an afternoon trip to Meadowhall, Alison, Anita or Mum could just take me in their cars. If I wanted to go out to the park on a sunny afternoon rather than sitting in the hospital gardens, we could. I even managed to surprise the children one afternoon when Alison and Mum wheeled me to the school gates to collect them at home time. I will never forget the way their faces lit up when they saw me in my wheelchair when they had been expecting Nana.

With every day out with the children I was beginning to feel like I was becoming more of a mum again. There were two main school events at the end of term in the middle of July and I was glad that I was physically well enough to make both of them.

The first was Woody's sports day, an event that could sometimes be a bit chaotic. But this year everything ran smoothly. Mark came to collect me from hospital and we drove to the sports field with our folding chairs, picnic blankets and food hampers. It was like being a proper family again as Mark wheeled my chair to the front of the field and there we decamped with our friends from the school run. I watched as Woody's team bounced to victory in the inflatable space hopper race. When it was time for the mum's race I would have given anything to join in instead of watching from the sidelines. But Woody was so pleased that I was there. He sat on my lap for most of the afternoon, which wasn't particularly comfy for either of us, but it meant we could be close.

My presence at India's school leavers' concert was less successful. India was moving up from junior to comprehensive school the next term and to mark the occasion the school always held a concert to say goodbye. It was a big occasion for India and Alison's daughter Charlotte, who were both in the leaver's class and singing in the concert. Mark's parents were in the audience along with Alison and Anita, whose children were also taking part. Alison wheeled me into the hall and put my brakes on at the end of a row, taking her seat next to me. The hall was packed with the proud parents and grandparents of all the children on stage. By now most people in the school knew of my situation and accepted my disability, so I was comfortable in their company.

The curtains opened, the audience fell silent, the music started and the concert began. Alison's daughter stepped onto the stage with her class to sing. Suddenly there was a loud noise from the audience and everyone turned to look in my direction. It sounded like someone was impersonating the donkey from the *Shrek* movies. It was me. Just at the moment when Charlotte had started singing, Alison had whispered to me, 'I don't know why Charlotte is doing this. She can't sing.' Childish I know, but I couldn't stop laughing. Anita, sitting near me, was horrified. Mark's parents in the row behind were mortified. India, who was sat in the wings waiting nervously for her moment on stage, wanted to die of embarrassment. The more I tried to stop myself laughing, the louder I laughed. And the louder I laughed, the more Alison laughed. But no one else was laughing. In the end Anita had to split Alison and I by sitting in between us, like we were a couple of naughty schoolgirls. When the concert was over, India was close to tears and refused to speak to me.

'You ruined my concert, I was so ashamed,' she cried on the way back to hospital in the back of the ambulance. I kept trying to apologise. Alison said sorry on my behalf, but she went into a total sulk. When we got back on to the ward Alison spoke to the nurses. 'Can you turn Kate's volume down? She's embarrassed herself this afternoon,' she joked. But India didn't find it funny.

Alone that night I was still laughing to myself about the concert. I hadn't laughed so much since before the stroke. I felt uplifted but also a bit guilty. I texted India with another apology and hoped that by the time I saw her again at the weekend she would have forgiven me, which she did.

With every trip out, I felt I was getting more independent. I was managing to stay out for longer from the initial couple of hours. I still could not walk more than a couple of steps without help, but I could transfer my body weight from the wheelchair to a car seat and I was managing a whole day sitting in the chair without feeling tired or uncomfortable. All this, I thought, must mean I would be able to go on holiday to Cornwall in a couple of weeks.

Chapter 31
Say my Name, Mum

FOR THE FIRST FIVE months I was in hospital, Mark had difficulty in coming to terms with the prognosis that I would never walk or talk again. It was hard for him to open up to his close family, so there was no chance he was going to offload his burdens on a work colleague or passing acquaintance. When people asked him how I was doing, as they often did, he would reply with a non-committal 'as well as can be expected'.

My speech therapist had told him I would never talk again. Even with the trachi out, I could not get the air I needed into my voice box to make my vocal chords work. I was not even trying to form words. In her experience this was a sign that I would never talk again. Therefore the therapy focussed on exercises that would at least help me to regain my swallowing techniques with the long-term goal of eating again.

While Mark could see progress with my movement and my muscle strength, he accepted the therapist's direct words, 'Kate will never speak again,' even if he could not bring himself to tell others. But he was forced to come out and admit this bad news one evening while he was out with some of his mountain-biking mates. He had been telling them how I was now standing on my own, writing and whizzing around the ward on an electric wheelchair. One of his friends said how great it would be to talk to me again.

'Kate will never talk again,' Mark said, and the shock registered on his friend's face. It was an important moment in Mark's healing process that he could actually admit the inevitable. So imagine his amazement when, within the space of forty-eight hours, I proved him and the therapist wrong.

It was a Friday night when I spoke my first words. Mark had brought the children in to see me and they were all in a good mood as they, like me, were counting down the days to their holidays. Seven more sleeps and they'd be going away; they were full of beans. I wanted to ask Woody if he had been to his piano lessons. India was holding my communication board so I started to spell out Woody's name. India pointed to the words and Harvey wrote it down, it was a process that took ten times longer than it should. On this particular night they were excitable and didn't have the patience for a laborious spelling session. Woody looked at me and asked, 'Why don't you just say it?' I didn't think I could. Up until that point I had made animal-like grunting noises, but nothing that sounded like words or that made any sense. My speech therapy was focussing on exercises that would strengthen my tongue in order to swallow and eat. No one thought I was capable of speaking.

But I like a challenge and Woody had set one. I thought of the mouth exercises I had been practising and tried to shape my mouth to form a word. 'Uugh!' I said. It sounded nothing like Woody. I tried again. 'Ood.' I was still grunting like a constipated pig. 'Give it your best shot, Kate,' the voice in my head was urging me on. 'Oody,' I said as I felt my tongue making new shapes inside my mouth.

Mark whose attention had been drifting off to the TV in the corner, suddenly turned to me in surprise.

'Kate, did you just say Woody?' I grinned smugly and said it over and over again, 'Oody, oody, oody.' Like a baby learning to speak, the words were only recognisable to those who knew what I was trying to say, but they were words and it proved I could get enough air into my voice box to form words. After Woody's name I tried India's which came out as 'Indi' and Harvey, which came out as 'Avvy'. Mark was ecstatic, he could eat his words; I could speak again.

All weekend I practised and practised, stringing one or two syllables together to form words. When my favourite nurse came on duty the following Monday morning to give me my usual dose of drugs, I said, 'Morning, Oliver'. He stopped in his tracks.

'Did you just speak?' he asked, hardly believing what he had heard.

'Morning, Oliver,' I said again, this time slower and more pronounced. He broke down and cried. 'I became a nurse, for moments like this,' he wept. I thought, you soft lump, you should be happy not crying.

Within minutes Sophie, my speech therapist, rushed down to my bedside to see what Oliver was making such a fuss about. 'Morning, Soph,' I said. She too started crying, astounded and also delighted to be proved wrong.

From that day on, my speech and language therapy took on a whole new importance. Sophie increased the exercises. In addition to the swallowing exercises, I had a new programme of oral motor exercises designed to strengthen my lips and develop the muscles at the back of my tongue in order to form words.

Gradually I began to speak in a monotone voice that Mark later called my 'stroke voice'. The initial surprise of those first words spoken soon wore off as I became more confident with my words. I was able to give him verbal grief as well as the stern stares.

Chapter 32
Don't Leave me Again

To SAY I WAS excited about my first holiday to Cornwall was an understatement; I was like a kid at Christmas, counting down the sleeps. Since the disappointment of having to stay in hospital for my birthday, I was determined that I would be fit enough.

I had worked extra hard at physio, pushed the boundaries and exhausted myself and my therapists with my continual drive for more. But as the day approached, it was becoming more and more obvious that I wasn't going to be allowed to make the three-hundred-mile journey. I had managed eight- or nine-hour days out but I had not yet built up to an overnight stay at home. My nursing team ruled that it was too far, for too long. I was absolutely gutted. As the departure date grew closer, I hoped they would make a dramatic U-turn or that Mark might change his mind and stay at home. I was spending more and more time with Mark and the children at weekends and was looking forward to having the chance to be together as a family.

The holiday was going ahead as planned. I was really pissed off. Not just because of my own disappointment but, I thought, why go so far away? Why not lose your deposit?' I knew that the children were looking forward to their summer holiday with Alison's family and our friends the Manion family again, but I needed them more. 'Please stay home,' I begged, 'we can rearrange something later as a family.' But he ignored me. And this hurt more than anything.

It also caused friction between Mark and my mum and Dave. They could see how angry and depressed I was getting and worried that I would undo all the good work I had made with my therapy. Dave and Mum suggested that Mark should cancel the holiday and stay close to home, where we could all go out for day trips. But they were going, end of story.

I went into such a major sulk I posted on Facebook, 'They've all gone away. I know they need a holiday but so many tests to my strength. I've lost trust and control in my life as well as my family.'

Like the previous holiday, they kept in touch with emails and phone calls, but it only upset me to hear them. For a few days after they had gone, I withdrew into my shell. I made no effort in my therapy sessions, I couldn't be bothered. I thought, what's the point if I'm never going to go back to a normal life?

Anita, Mum and my other friends rallied round with visits, but I couldn't be bothered with small talk. Mum was so worried that she had a word with my psychotherapist who tried to get me to talk my way out of my depression with positive thoughts. 'What was I missing?' That was easy: my family and my fitness. 'Where would I rather be?' I told her I wished I could be high in the Peak District running across the bridle paths as I had done so regularly in my old life. My psychologist thought it might help if she made me a meditation CD. She recorded herself talking about the Peak District. Her gentle, calming voice described the views over the villages, the smells of the countryside and the adrenalin rush of running downhill. For an hour

I sat in bed, listening to her voice floating in and out of my conscience, imagining myself out pounding across the hills. It did the trick, I felt calmer and happier. Until she insisted on making me listen to it every day for ever more and I soon got bored with it. I came to dread the bloody meditation CD and hid it in the back of my locker.

Eventually I came out of my mood and threw myself back into my therapy with renewed energy. I was determined that Mark would see even more of a difference when he came back from holidays. I signed up for every session going, including book club and music therapy. The music therapy made me feel like a right dork, wobbling my head to bang a tambourine in time to a pre-recorded music track or playing a keyboard with a laser by breaking the beam with my head movements, but at least these sessions got me off the ward for an extra hour a week.

The book club was run by a volunteer from outside who came in once a week for those of the Osborn 4 patients who were able to read and discuss their books. In my old life I had enjoyed going to book club which had been more of a gossip session than a literary salon. We had ten to twelve members, all fellow mums, who took turns to meet up at one another's houses. We voted on a book we all wanted to read, sometimes it would be a crime thriller or a personal memoir. The next month we discussed the book. I have to admit the actual book discussion took all of ten minutes; the rest of the night was taken over by wine and whinging about our kids and husbands. During my time in hospital the book club actually became vital for Alison, Jaqui and Anita, who used it as it should be … a forum to discuss books. They chose memoirs of other stroke patients, *The Diving Bell and the Butterfly*, Hasso and Catherine von Breddow's

In The Blink of an Eye. Both these books were depressing to my friends as both authors never recovered from their locked-in syndrome and died. Yet they were able to understand the frustrations of a locked-in patient. From reading these books and discussing them in book club they were able to gain a practical insight into caring for someone with locked-in syndrome. When I was still locked in in the ICU these books gave them the inspiration to come up with the blinking and pain charts as a means to help me express myself.

I too read Bauby's book *The Diving Bell and the Butterfly*, which Alison had given me with a cautious recommendation. I was deeply affected by the tragedy of the French journalist who, like me, was locked in his own body. The author never recovered from the condition which he described as like being inside an old-fashioned deep-sea diving suit with a brass helmet, while his spirit remained free as a butterfly. By sheer force of willpower and determination, he had painstakingly blinked every single letter of the book to his editor. The book became not only his legacy to the world but, having been made into an award-winning film, it also brought the terrifying situation of a person with locked-in syndrome to a wider audience. Reading his book I understood and empathised with Bauby's mistrust of the medical profession, his levels of resentment and anger and his joy at seeing his children. This book also proved to me that I had a story with more to offer and I started scribbling down the notes for my own version. Unlike Bauby I could not, and would not, allow my imagination to run away with me. In my mind imagination was an indulgence, and time spent daydreaming of how things once were, and might never be again, only distracted me from the road ahead –

getting better.

Without Mark and the children, the week seemed to drag but when they came home I was so pleased to see them the anger I had melted away. I had some good news for them too, I was being allowed out for my first overnight visit the following weekend. It was the beginning of the end, home was on the horizon.

Chapter 33
Why am I Fighting a Constant Battle?

SOMETIMES I FELT LIKE my recovery was one continual fight: me against the medical profession. On these occasions I thought of myself as Hollywood boxing champ Rocky. As a child I had loved the *Rocky* films, partly because I had a huge schoolgirl crush on Sylvester Stallone. On days when all the odds seemed stacked against me I would pretend I was underdog fighter Rocky Balboa in the black corner, and the might of the Northern General Hospital's medical experts were Apollo Creed, the heavyweight champion, in the red corner. I would hum the Rocky theme in my head, pushing me on to victory.

There were many battles along the way as I began counting down the days to my first overnight home visit and the weeks to my final release. With all the medical tests to pass, and procedures to follow, all the odds seemed to be stacked against me; every day I felt like I was playing a waiting game. I was battling with my doctors and therapists, who had other patients in their care, and could not accept my urgency to get things done. As the clock ticked, every day I spent waiting for a specialist to look at test results, or give orders, was a day less of the rest of my life. As the days dragged, I became demotivated and I just wanted to go home.

I already had a plan. I had been in contact with the manager of my local Esporta leisure club in Sheffield via email and asked him to help me run again. I put together a business case, 'if you give me free membership and help me to run by Christmas, it will be good publicity for your gym.' The manager was receptive to my proposal. His own father had suffered a stroke which had left him bitter and sad before his death, so he was supportive of my determination to get one hundred per cent fit. During one of my day trips out of the hospital, Alison took me down to meet him and we agreed on a long-term fitness programme. With this in mind, the hospital's physiotherapy seemed slow and laborious and I just wanted to move on.

I wanted to be able to control my bladder without the need for a catheter. I wanted to be able to walk upstairs to the bathroom at home and I demanded to have my PEG taken out. None of these things would have prevented my release from hospital from a medical point of view. I had read about some poor sods who never came out of locked-in syndrome. They had their houses converted into a home-hospital ward so that they could go back to living with their families. But I didn't want this for my family, I wanted to be as normal as I could and I was adamant that I would go home to the house that I had left behind, not a special-needs conversion. Our house had been modernised and had a wide, open hallway and a large open-plan kitchen diner and toilet downstairs, which offered easy access for a wheelchair. But the contentious point was the bathroom.

My occupational therapist had recommended that Mark should convert our ground-floor garage into a new bathroom as stairs were a huge obstacle for me, and installing a stairlift was out of the question because of the layout of our house. But I didn't want any special adaptations; I didn't want my house to be any different from my friends' homes. It probably says more about my prejudices than anything else, but the thought of having a house which said, 'disabled person lives here,' was abhorrent to me. Don't get me wrong, I know that no disabled person wants to be dependent on others or have to rely on specially adapted toilets and wide doors for their wheelchairs. I appreciated that all these adaptations can make life easier for the patient but I did not want them.

'Want to walk upstairs to bathroom,' I scrawled on a sheet of paper which I handed to my occupational therapist. 'In time. Let's concentrate on getting you walking on the flat first,' came the reply. It was not the answer I wanted. She had thrown down the gauntlet: I would walk upstairs.

This sheet of paper became my mantra, I stuck it on my locker as a daily reminder to my therapists and carers and even my family that I had set a new goal for myself.

One afternoon when I was on a home visit with Dave, I persuaded him to take me upstairs. At first he was reluctant and made all kinds of excuses, but I nagged him and eventually he gave in. I stood at the bottom of our stairs looking up to the top. I imagined I was at the base camp of Mount Kilimanjaro and the fourteen steps in front of me were the final push to the summit. With the Rocky theme playing in my head, I put my total trust in Dave and held on to the handrail to pull myself up. Dave stood behind me, holding my hips and moved my legs one stair at a time in tandem with his. Even with my fragile weight it was hard work. One push, then we stopped on the next step before pressing ahead. Two steps, stop. Three, then on until half an hour later we were at the top. I sat down exhausted but delighted. I had done it and no one could take away my huge sense of happiness at achieving something that everyone thought was out of my reach. I swore Dave to secrecy and said nothing, not even to Mark, who was contemplating taking the medical advice and using the money left over from the charity bike ride to build a downstairs bathroom in our garage.

A week later I was sitting with the nurses at their central desk when I felt the need to confess all.

'What would you say if I told you I had walked upstairs?' I asked the 'Drill Sergeant'. I had recently started working with the 'Sergeant' who had been brought in to cover when my main physiotherapist went on maternity leave. I was fond of the Drill Sergeant, he was competitive and driven like me, and he pushed me harder and gave me more goals, hence his nickname. 'I'd say you would be lying, wouldn't you?' he replied.

I laughed mischievously – and he realised I was telling the truth. Boy, did he tear me off a strip.

'I can't believe you could be so irresponsible,' he warned. 'Do you realise how much danger you were putting yourself and Dave in? What if you had fallen? One slip up and you could have undone all the good progress you've made …' On and on he droned so, like a naughty child, I blocked out his words. I had done it and I was proud. A week later the Drill Sergeant and my occupational therapist took me home and I walked the stairs officially.

That first official ascent was slow and considered. Using a crutch to support my left side, holding on to the handrail of the banister with my stronger right side, with my physiotherapist's hands around my waist to steady me, I pushed up one step at a time, tentatively at first then building in confidence as I neared the top. I had managed to climb the small flight of four stairs on the

Osborn 4 ward three times so I was confident I could do it. With my therapists and Mark watching I was worried I would fail, but I succeeded. When night came, Mark and I were alone to make the final ascent.

Once it was agreed that I could manage the stairs, I had won the battle over the bathroom. But the next round was the time-frame. Mark and the occupational therapists agreed that we needed to convert the bathroom into a wet/shower room to make it easier for me to walk into. We would use the money left over from the bike ride to make this conversion. I could see their logic, but I couldn't accept how long it would take.

'I've found a plumber who can do the bathroom,' Mark announced one evening, looking rather pleased with himself. It was no ordinary job and he had been struggling to find a tradesman who was willing to undertake such a specialist project. 'But they say we will have to wait three months to get the materials shipped in from Europe.

This news was no use to me when I was desperate to go home. Both Mark and the therapists agreed it would be better for me to wait in hospital than to go home to a building site. 'Get someone else who can do it quicker,' I argued, becoming more and more impatient.

'But I've been trying, Kate. I've been through Yellow Pages and none of the local plumbers will touch it. This plumber is a specialist, he knows what he's doing. Honestly, Kate, I'm doing everything I can do get it done as soon as we can,' Mark reasoned. No one seemed to understand my urgency. I was getting paranoid that Mark might not want me home, a flashback to my first review returned to haunt me. Eventually he managed to persuade the plumber to juggle jobs, put pressure on the suppliers to treat our order with urgency and work started. But it was still too slow for my liking.

I wrote on my Facebook page:

It's cruel not letting me be at home with my family because we are having a new bathroom. I know Mark feels responsible but it's just not fair

As this fight was going on at home, in hospital I was going through potty training for adults. 'Flip flowing,' was the method of training the muscles in the bladder to work again which, if successful, would eventually lead to the removal of the catheter. After almost eight months of non-use, the muscles were slack. The nurses would flip the switch on the catheter tube down to stop the urine flowing into the bag.

This had the effect that urine would build up in my bladder, then the nurses would flip the switch back on and it would rush out into the bag again. Sometimes this resulted in a 'by-pass' where the urine leaked out and ran down the side of the tube. I could feel it happening but was powerless to stop it. This process went on for over a month, building up from thirty minutes to four hours and as my muscles became stronger and my movement improved in my arm, I was able to switch the flow on and off myself. When I was able to hold my wee for four hours, the nurses started allowing me to go to the toilet. At the same time I was also being retrained to use my bowels which, just like a toddler, resulted in more accidents than success. I had to retrain my body to recognise the signs that I needed to go, and then get there and get my trousers down before it was too late. Going to the toilet required two nurses to hoist me into my electric wheelchair so I could drive myself to the cubicle, where they would help me out other end. This was a lengthy process and I didn't always succeed in making it in time. Fortunately the nurses gave me thick incontinence pads to catch the flow. One afternoon I was sitting on my bed, practising this flip-flowing and waiting for the nurses to take me to the toilet when I thought it would be a laugh to text Alison, 'Call me Tena lady'. 'I will not call you Tena lady,' came back her adamant reply she could not appreciate how I needed to be able to make fun of myself for my own sanity.

With the catheter tube, my agenda and the doctor's timescale were again at odds. Once I had been to the toilet regularly I wanted it out. It was another sign of illness that I didn't need. The nurses however didn't see the rush as it made life easier for them not having to take me to the toilet every couple of hours. I insisted, but nothing was done. Luckily for me the catheter removal came by accident one Sunday night when one of the nurses was injecting drugs into my PEG and accidentally pulled the tube out. It bloody stung, but I didn't complain. It was out and there was no way it was going back in. She confessed her mistake to the ward manager, who wanted to put it back in. 'No way,' I said. 'Will go to toilet.' Many restless nights and soggy pad moments followed as my bladder was put to the test. Even now my mum I is convinced that I pulled it out myself, but I didn't. It was an accident. It took longer than a month before I was managing to get to the toilet successfully all the time. The day I was allowed to discard the nappies and wear knickers was a great leap forward. Without the bulky pads I felt slimmer and freer to move around.

I had another major fight with my nutritionist, a strict woman who was a right jobsworth. Our relationship started to go downhill after my painful constipation episode when she refused to accept that my diet was a contributing factor and I was convinced it was.

She was determined that I should put on weight by continuing with the liquid food ingested into my stomach instead of proper food. My feeding times took place during the night when I was hooked up to a liquid feed which trickled into my PEG. That way my drip didn't get in the way of therapy sessions. I never once had proper food at meal times and generally I didn't mind as my family and friends would never be so thoughtless as to eat in front of me. The only time it ever became an issue was one evening when Mark came to visit straight from work and had just finished eating a packet of crisps. His cheese and onion breath was unbearable and made me realise how much I missed my favourite salt and vinegar crisps.

For me the PEG was the last obvious sign that I was an invalid. Once I had succeeded with the spoon and water trials I decided that I was ready to drink tea.

During one of these swallow trials, Sophie the therapist said 'Yorkshire or Earl Grey?' As if she needed to ask. 'Earl Grey, please,' I replied. Off she went to the kitchen to put the kettle on and came back with a beaker half full of milky Earl Grey. Handing it to me, she watched with pride as I held the plastic cup in my right hand and drank, sucking the liquid through the spout in the lid. No words could describe that moment as I drank my first cup of tea. I was in control. The ping-pong ball exercises were working, I was able to suck the liquid into my mouth. I didn't need a nurse to spoon-feed me tiny drops of tea. I was drinking on my own and it felt good. I drained every single drop out of that beaker. 'Any chance of seconds?' I asked, with a cheeky grin.

'Don't push your luck. Maybe tomorrow.' It was the reply I had been expecting.

From this I progressed to pureed food, yoghurt and

large bars of Cadbury's Caramel chocolate, which my visitors brought in and hid in my locker. I would put a chunk on my tongue and allow it to melt, the sweet stickiness slipping down my throat. I had learnt to eat slowly, tilting my head downwards, taking very small mouthfuls so that the food would pass down my gullet. This generally went well, although there were some occasions when food got stuck in my pipe. As I had no coughing or gagging reflex I could not voluntarily eject it, so one of the nurses showed me a clever, although completely unorthodox, trick. They would tickle the back of my throat with my toothbrush and I automatically coughed up the food. This technique came in handy after I left hospital. The food seemed to be going down the right way and over time I had gained two stone in weight. It had reached a point where my PEG was only being used to administer painkillers and my daily dose of liquid cod liver oil. While I was in hospital I was happy to continue taking my drugs this way as the cod liver oil tasted so foul that I was convinced I could taste it as it went directly into my stomach. Eventually my nutritionist could see she was fighting a losing battle to stop me eating. She made me sign a disclaimer admitting that I was going against her advice but I didn't mind, I was managing my own nutrition and gained a stone on my choccy caramel and soup diet.

Before I could have the PEG taken out Ming the Merciless had to give his approval and for that to happen I had to pass another videofluoroscopy. I flatly refused to go through this again. Having already failed two I didn't want the mental pressure of building myself up to be disappointed. I also did not want my body to undergo a third dose of radiation in three months. The week before I was due to go home, the PEG nurse came to tell me how to use my PEG once I got home. 'Piss off, I'm not taking it home,' was my curt reply. I dug my heels in and eventually they came round to my way of thinking. Four days before I left hospital one of the junior doctors came to pull it out and it really hurt. It reminded me of pulling an elephant through the eye of a needle as the rubber bumper which was fitted inside my stomach to hold the PEG in place had to be pulled out through a hole one fifth its size. With no anaesthetic, just a dose of paracetamol (the final feeding through my PEG) I could feel every tug and turn as the doctor pulled. With a final pop it was out. 'That didn't hurt me one bit,' the doc said. It took a while as the pain subsided before I could see the funny side. He warned me that it night take twenty-four hours for the hole to start healing under the dressing and in the meantime I felt like a character from *Tom and Jerry* with a hole in my middle.

I recall how I even had to fight for a blood transfusion when I discovered I was anaemic. I had been suffering heavier and heavier blood flows during my periods, when in hospital. Ever since I had given birth to India I had always suffered heavy periods. At their worst I was forced to stay indoors some days as I was too embarrassed to go out. Occasionally it would drain me of my energy, but I had lived with it for more than ten years, and when I was a fully functioning, able-bodied woman I was able to cope. When I was dependent on nurses to change my bloodied incontinence pads, it became even more noticeable. On this particular day, 'Sara Short' came to change my nappy and was horrified by the amount of blood I had lost. 'My God, Kate, you look like you've been attacked!' she exclaimed as she cleaned me up and tried to restore my dignity. It was hugely degrading. After medical investigations it was decided that I should have a coil fitted to control the blood loss. For this procedure I was taken to the gynaecology wing of the hospital and had the device fitted. It had the desired effect, from that point on my periods became lighter and more manageable. But I still didn't feel right. My limited amount of energy was draining from me so quickly that I even had to miss physiotherapy one morning because I was just worn out.

I knew my body and to me there was something very wrong. When Mark came to visit me I asked him to hand me a mirror. Looking at my reflection, I pulled down my lower eyelid and was shocked to see white translucent skin instead of healthy, pink arteries. After Mark had gone home and the ward had closed its doors to visitors, I wheeled myself out to the nurses' desk to show the nurses my discovery. Blood tests revealed I was severely anaemic. My red blood cell count was six when it should have been twelve. No amount of iron tablets would have been able to increase the count quickly enough, so Ming the Merciless ruled I should have a blood transfusion.

This should not have been such a big deal, considering everything I had already been through. But I got nervous when the night staff on the ward confessed they had not given a blood transfusion in twenty years. Fortunately they decided the transfusion would have to wait until the following morning when one of the nurses from the blood bank could show them what to do. Next morning, as the two pints of donor blood dripped into my veins, I could not help thinking of all the scare stories I had heard in the news about blood infected with HIV and hepatitis being given to patients with haemophilia and I went into an irrational panic. But there was nothing I could do, I needed the blood and the transfusion worked wonderfully well.

As I watched the alien blood trickling into my body I was reminded of a film night I had had with Alison and India when India had brought in her favourite *Twilight* film. The three of us had settled down in the visitors' lounge – although it was no substitute for curling up on the sofa at home it was a break from being on the ward. As she put the disc in the player, India said 'It's a film about vampires, Mum. Do you know what vampires are?' Alison was quick to jump to my defence saying 'Of course she knows what vampires are. Your mum has had a stroke, but she's not stupid.'

Chapter 34
Home for the Weekend

I HAD BEEN LOOKING forward to spending my first night at home, free from nurses and hospital routines. I wanted to be in my own environment, making my own rules, staying up late, eating when and what I wanted. But within a short time of arriving home, I realised what a pressure cooker of stress our family life had become. Harvey and Woody were back to their old games, fighting and arguing, just as they had been when I checked out almost eight months earlier. Mark was shouting at them to behave. Good grief, have I landed in a war zone? I thought.

Without my catheter I could use the toilet like a normal person, but because of the slowness of movement, which Mark often compared to a robot, I had to plan ahead so I would not embarrass myself and be caught short. We had a small toilet off our kitchen and I had been given a frame which fitted around it and allowed me to lower myself onto the toilet seat. However I needed help from Mark to pull down my trousers and ease me gently onto the seat. Once seated I was safe, but Mark could not relax, he was worried I'd use the washbasin to pull myself back up to standing position, even though he had told me not to. So he was constantly hovering around the door, which did not make for the most relaxing of toilet breaks.

Later that evening we settled down to watch Saturday night television as a family. Woody snuggled up close to me for the hugs he had waited almost eight months for.

'I've missed you, Mum,' he whispered in my ear as put his arm lightly around my body. He was afraid of hurting me or, worse still, accidentally pulling out my PEG, which was the way my drugs were fed through my stomach. Our cuddles didn't last for long as my jumpy legs went and spoiled the moment.

At 7 every night, without fail, my legs would start twitching and aching, with what was commonly called Restless Leg Syndrome. I had first suffered with the condition when I was in the final month of pregnancy with India and again when I was having Harvey and Woody. On those occasions I was at least able to walk around the room with my bump to ease the discomfort. Now it was thought that my restless legs were another symptom caused by the disruption to the pathways in my brain which usually ensured smooth muscle movements. Ironically the post locked-in condition was made more unbearable because I couldn't simply get out of bed and walk around the room. In hospital this, along with my general insomnia, made for many long and boring nights. At home at last I had hoped for some relief but it was not to be. I could not sit and watch TV, so like every other night, I went to bed early and lay down. Mark was there to help me up the stairs as he had been earlier in the week when the physio team had helped me. But now we were on our own and we managed pretty well.

Going to bed took some preparation. Just like being in hospital I had to regulate my liquid intake, 7.30 being the cut off point for my last cup of tea. It might seem that I was obsessed by the toilet routine and I was. I had a fear of having to get up in the middle of the night to use the toilet. Being in bed without a nurse on the end of a buzzer, I felt vulnerable and scared. Our bedroom was thirty-six steps up in the loft, so Mark and I decided we would sleep in Harvey's room, which was only fifteen steps up to the first floor, and Harvey would have our bed. When my head hit the pillow that first night an overwhelming sense of calm and relief rushed over me. The softness of a feather pillow; the smell of freshly laundered cotton pillowcases under my head instead of the stiff, starchy hospital issue; even the sensation of having a duvet to gently caress my body instead of the tightly drawn hospital blankets was a treat. 'I could get used to this, quite quickly,' I thought to myself as I drifted off into the deepest sleep I had had since coming out of the coma.

Mark, though, had a less comfortable night. He was constantly aware of rolling over and squashing me and consequently slept lightly and kept to his side of the bed for fear of hurting me.

*   *   *

During my occupational therapy sessions, my therapist had been preparing me for independent living, those simple things we take for granted like making a cup of tea or baking cakes. These sessions, which took place in a small kitchen on the ward above Osborn 4, were great fun as I relearned to switch on the kettle without scalding myself and to bake cakes following a recipe. This was a totally new area for me, as I have never followed a recipe in my life. I'm more of a throw it in a bowl and hope for the best type of cook, and this method has always served me well, particularly with my flapjacks, which were the pride of the PTA. While my therapist was carefully weighing out the flour and sugar,

216

I would be throwing the ingredients together with some limited success. My drop scones were delicious but my flapjacks were a disaster, I think we left them in the oven too long and they turned into rock cakes. After baking we cleared up and I sampled my home-cooking, which was a real treat, and take the leftovers back to the ward for my visitors. It reminded me of those days I would come home from school home-economics lessons and subject my mother and Dave to some charcoaled creation that started life as an apple crumble. *Just made scones and washed up. Don't want to make a habit of it'* I announced on Facebook after one of my lessons. On other days we made soup, which I would also eat. I wasn't supposed to but my therapist had given up trying to stop me as I became more determined to do what I wanted.

At home that first weekend I was able to put my skills from the hospital kitchen into practice as we cooked our first Sunday roast dinner as a family. Mark prepared the chicken for the roasting pan, India peeled the potatoes, Harvey chopped up the broccoli and carrots and Woody and I supervised from my wheelchair. I firmly believe in the importance of sitting down as a family to eat, which was one of the things Mark always insisted the grandparents did in my absence. Just being part of the activity made me feel human again. When lunch was ready we all sat around the table and the rest of the family helped themselves. My dinner had been blitzed in the food processor so it looked like baby food, but boy did it taste good. As I fed myself, I savoured every gravy-rich, chicken-blended mouthful. It felt so good to be back at the heart of the family.

From this successful one-nighter, my home visits became a regular event, building up to two nights.

These trips were designed to help me become less institutionalised and give my family a taste of what lay ahead. After a couple of weeks I was becoming more independent in attitude. Back on the ward I was also promoted to my own private, single-bed room, with my own hand basin and wardrobe. It was further away from the nurse's station and it meant that I was getting closer to going home. During this period of my recovery, I was saddened to hear of the death of Alison's dad. In May Alison had told me he had been diagnosed with brain cancer and throughout my rehabilitation, Alison had been keeping me upbeat and positive, while she had been dealing with her own personal tragedy. Alison and her dad had been close, and it upset me that I was physically unable to be her shoulder to cry on when she needed it most. I was determined I would attend the funeral out of loyalty and support to Alison.

On the day of the funeral service one of Alison's friends took me in my wheelchair to Dore church. The church was full, her dad was a retired businessman in Dore and well-known and respected in the community. Up until that point I had not given a thought to how I would react to being so close to death again. As we sat in the church waiting for the funeral procession, one of the villagers tapped me on the shoulder and asked how I was feeling. 'I'm fine,' I said in my slow stroke voice and then, for no reason whatsoever, I started to laugh. At that moment the organist stopped to turn the page of her music book and everyone heard my donkey laugh. I was so embarrassed for myself and everyone there, I knew it was out of order but it was a nervous laugh and I could not help myself. I was making an inappropriate braying noise when the coffin entered the church. Later I felt I had to apologise to Alison for what seemed like disrespect to her family, but it was just my unsettled reaction to the funeral. I had not expected to be so moved as tributes were paid to her dad. But as I looked at the coffin laid out in wreaths, I imagined myself inside. I pictured a wreath with *Mum* on the casket and a heartbroken Mark, India, Harvey and Woody standing beside it. Tearfully, I looked around at the sombre faces of the mourners and wondered, who would have been at my funeral?

Chapter 35
I Know I'm Not a Good Patient

TWO WEEKS BEFORE I left hospital I had my final specialist therapy assessment. It read...

'Mrs Allatt has demonstrated a tremendous fortitude in driving forward her rehabilitation from an initially poor prognosis to her current considerable recovery. However this drive has also inclined her to take unnecessary risks and ignore advice from therapists on occasion which needs to be monitored whilst not unfairly restricting her progress.'

There it was in black and white, I was not a good patient. This I already knew and quite frankly as I have said before, I didn't care. In reaction to this I posted on Facebook:

I am not impulsive, I do however take considered risks.

I knew my body better than anyone. All the doctors, nurses and therapists may have spent years in medical school, swotting up on case studies and biology and physiology text books, but they didn't know me. I had spent forty years in my body, I knew what signs to look for when I was ill, like the anaemia incident, and I knew how much therapy and exercise my body could withstand, which was always more than average. I wasn't a text-book case. I did not want specialist treatment but I wanted to be treated as an individual and this was the root of many of my ongoing battles with the nursing staff.

I was marked out as a rule-breaker within days of transferring to Osborn 4 when I was given sponge lolly sticks soaked in apple juice to freshen my mouth. Being so poorly I was not allowed any liquid but one of the nurses took pity on me and my parched mouth. She brought a carton of apple juice and dipped the sponge into the liquid before dabbing it on my tongue to take away the stale dryness. This was bliss and as soon as she turned her back, Alison continued to feed me this juice. In no time the carton was empty, I had been sucking it down into my lungs when it was only meant to refresh the inside of my mouth. The nurses had to get the lung hoover to suck the juice out and the sponge lollipops were taken away.

It was the first of many privileges I abused. In the early days when I was allowed to be pushed outside in my wheelchair, I would encourage my visitors to take me outside the perimeter of the ward and garden. I remember putting one poor nurse in a panic when he turned to look for us and we had disappeared. Even in the weeks leading up to my discharge I caused the nurses a headache by staying out late. If I was due to return at 4 p.m., I would quite often call and tell them, 'I'm staying overnight' see you in the morning.'

One night after I had been moved to the private ward I got my neck wedged in the cot bars and had to use my mobile phone to call for help. I was reaching out to press the buzzer to call a nurse to take me to the loo; the call button had been put back on the wall behind my bed and in overstretching I got stuck with the metal railings digging into my windpipe. Too weak to lift myself back up, I dangled there helplessly. Luckily my mobile phone was on the bed next to my hand with the ward's phone number programmed into it, so I managed to press the number on my mobile to call front desk for help. When Oliver answered, a pathetic breathless voice on the other end said, 'It's Kate, I need help.' He looked up from his desk and came to my rescue.

I also had a short fuse when it came to student nurses. Northern General was the main teaching hospital for the area and every six weeks there was a new batch of students learning from the staff and patients on Osborn 4. I hated being a guinea pig as everything took four times as long when you were in the hands of a trainee nurse. They were given the shitty jobs of changing my nappy or taking me to the toilet or shower so my indignity was prolonged through their lack of experience. I hated being watched by two or three pairs of eyes as my bottom was cleaned and changed. Even a straightforward trip to the shower took ages when the students were in charge. There was only one student nurse whom I ever took to and that was because she painted my nails and pampered me, and came into my private room and told me jokes, all the other used to piss me off. Eventually as my patience began to wear thin I told Sara Short to stop sending me students.

Another time I had been left on my own to shower when I lost my balance reaching out for my shampoo. The nurse would wheel me into the shower, put the brakes on my chair, help me to steady myself in a standing position and allow me to wash myself. When I finished I rang the buzzer and they collected me. This day, without thinking, I misjudged the distance between me and the shampoo bottle as I reached for it without thinking. I missed and lost my balance. My right hand couldn't move fast enough to save myself, I fell in slow motion, my head hitting the ground with a bang. I pulled the emergency chord and the nurses came to pick me up, blaming me for pushing the boundaries. But it was a genuine accident, which made me realise that I wasn't as independent as I liked to think. Yet I still refused to use the shower chair, preferring to take my chances and stand.

A week after the shower incident I was shaken by another fall as I was getting myself out of bed and into the electric wheelchair. My legs buckled under me and as I lunged to grab on to the bedside table, that too moved further away. My nose took the full impact as it hit the corner of the table and blood spurted out. I looked a sorry state when the nurses came to pick me up off the floor. The fall left me shaken and subdued. Later I wrote on Facebook:

'Oh dear another fall. Gave myself a bloody nose, but didn't straighten it'

Despite being the patient from hell, I formed a strong bond with several of the full-time nurses on the ward, who came to treat me as one of them, probably because I spent so much time on their workstation computer. One of the nurses I had most respect for was Running Man, maybe it was because he was a fellow runner that I struck a bond with him early on. I also discovered that he had an encyclopaedic brain and spent many an hour picking it, asking him what I needed to do to get rid of my catheter and nappies. He explained what I needed to do to be able to walk again. His advice was invaluable in helping speed up my recovery. Some of the younger nurses came into my private ward and would watch TV or use my computer. Even the ones I had disliked at the start for their fussiness and strictness, I eventually warmed to. I began to see them as friends rather than carers and they appreciated my straight-talking, positive attitude. Often I wheeled myself down to the nurses' staffroom and sat with them. One afternoon I was sitting with the nurses during their lunch break when the gay nurse started his usual moaning about his weight and how none of his diets ever seemed to work. As he spread his latest 'slimmer's lunch' of two packets of crisps, a chocolate bar and a WeightWatchers quiche out on the table, I wrote on a bit of paper, *Why don't you just eat less?* Oliver, who was sat listening to the conversation but not taking part, fell about laughing at my directness.

By the time I was ready to leave Osborn 4, I had experienced the good and bad side of the NHS nursing system and come to many conclusions. So as a parting gift I would like to offer my advice for doctors caring for cognitively-aware patients.

Don't assume that because I am unable to move, I am stupid. Try a simple blink test with the patient to establish brain power.

Don't talk around the patients, talk to them. Do you know how rude and frightening this is? Even if the patients can't talk back, they can understand what you are saying.

Do make eye contact. When your eyes are your only form of communication, to avoiding looking a patient in the eye is just plain ignorant.

Do make an effort to treat the root cause not just the symptoms. Is the patient in pain? If a simple action like moving a leg or a shoulder can relieve that pain, do it.

Don't assume that night-time is easy. It's the hardest time. Is your patient dreading the night time because he or she can't sleep? Find out promptly and give sleeping pills if necessary. Tiredness makes you feel worse than you already are.

Don't treat the patient as another case study. Remember each person is an individual and will have his or her own levels of pain tolerance and know what feels wrong.

Don't assume locked-in patients are crying because they are sad. It might just be a cry for help because they are too hot, too cold, or need turning. So don't ignore them hoping they'll eventually shut up.

Don't be pessimistic, be open-minded. Just because you do not have a positive experience of treating locked-in syndrome doesn't mean it can't happen. Read other people's positive stories and share them with the patients to give them real hope. Let them make up their own minds.

Don't ignore your patients' intuition. Remember they know their bodies better than you do.

Do something as simple as changing the TV channel for the patient. This doesn't require a degree in medicine but can have a positive impact on relieving the patient's boredom.

Don't limit the therapy; if a patient wants more let him or her have it.

Do not put barriers in place that block progress or limits or timescales on what should be achieved. Do listen, learn and encourage and set clearly defined goals every six weeks to keep the momentum going.

Don't give false hope, but do allow the patient to have hope. Negativity is more debilitating than the actual stroke.

Chapter 36
I Really Should Appreciate Mark More

IF THE NURSES THOUGHT I was the patient from hell, they could at least go home at the end of the day and switch off. Oliver, my favourite nurse, later told me that, in all his years of nursing, he had never encountered a patient with as much drive and determination to get better. Poor Mark had no respite from my incessant demands; he was my mouthpiece. No matter how unreasonable I was being he couldn't tell me that. He was caught between a rock and a hard place.

When I wanted my trachi out, Mark was the one I insisted should go and ask. He came back to my bed, avoiding my eyes with his, because he knew a 'no way' would make me mad. Behind the scenes Mark was getting blasted from all sides. The doctors explained that they were reluctant to take the trachi out too soon because it was not a straightforward job to reinsert it if my breathing failed. It would have meant a major operation and the risks far outweighed the benefits. Mark could understand their logic but he could not make me see reason.

'I KNOW MY OWN BODY. WHY WON'T ANYONE LISTEN TO ME?' I wrote out in angry letters. There was no easy answer. I always knew when Mark had bad news for me as he was unusually quiet.

With hindsight I can now see that he was in an impossible position but at the time I just thought, 'Why don't you grow a pair?'

Similarly when I wanted to have my feeding PEG removed, Mark was the one on the receiving end of my frustration. He later confessed that it seemed that everything he did was wrong. He was in a no-win situation. Even something as simple as asking a nurse to come and 'hoover' the saliva out of my mouth became a bone of contention. I would ask him to fetch a nurse and off he'd go.

'They are dealing with another patient, they'll be with you in a minute,' he explained.

I WANT THEM NOW. YOU ARE NOT HELPING ME, was my response. He would sigh and wander off in search of another helper.

When I got on to Facebook Mark signed up too, just so that he could keep in touch when he was at work. But this also ended in tears as I would continue our arguments online. We became a real-life soap opera and some friends later confessed they enjoyed reading our not-so-private marital tiffs.

They say you always hurt the one you love and that was certainly the case with Mark. All the anger and frustration that was building up inside me, which came from spending my life in a hospital bubble, was directed at him. Any lesser man might have walked away, but not Mark. When the going got tough, he just absorbed everything like a sponge, protecting me from my own prognosis and holding everything together. Never once did he shirk his nightly visit, he just put on a brave face and got on with it. Back home he was also getting grief from my mum, who quite often fought my corner, but Mark stood his ground, believing what he was doing was always for the right reason, even if the holiday to

Cornwall and the delay in getting the bathroom ready led to more stress. He often referred to himself as the 'donkey' there to do all the work like pulling up my trousers and helping me tie my trainer laces, while everyone else had the fun visits.

At my most unreasonable, Alison thought it necessary to jump to Mark's defence with a, 'Be nice to Mark. He's trying really hard.' When this happened I became even more incensed and it took months before I fully appreciated the sacrifices he had made and hard work he put in just to keep our family running as close to normal as possible.

Just a few days before I was discharged, Mark came to visit me and for the first time since February he was struck by how 'normal' I looked. I lay on the bed in the private room, unaware of his presence, fidgeting to get my legs comfortable. For a few minutes Mark remained out of sight just watching me in silence, feeling as proud as the day our first child was born. I felt his eyes on me and with a blunt, 'What the hell are you staring at?' broke the moment.

Chapter 37
I Have Served my Time, Thank You and Goodbye

I WAS GIVEN A release date. September 29 2010. I started counting the sleeps before I would be back in my own bed. It was a week earlier than expected but I had dug my heels in and demanded that I be allowed to go home. Mark was working in Germany, his parents were looking after the children, and the bathroom was still a building site. But I didn't care, I wanted to go home. Before Mark had left for his business trip we had a massive row in hospital. In the end I told him, 'Sort it out, I'm coming home.' There was no negotiation, I wanted to get out.

With Mark abroad, it was left to my mum to collect me from hospital. But before I could leave there was one final obstacle – the walk from my bed to the ward entrance. Two months earlier I had written a message to Oliver saying, 'I will walk out of here.' At the time he rolled his eyes as if to say, 'we'll see'.

On the morning of my discharge my mum was on video camera duty to record my marathon effort. I had set myself this final goal and I had to succeed. There was no pressure from the nurses and therapists, they would have happily wheeled me to the car and waved me off, but I wanted to prove to myself that I could do it.

To prepare for my grand finale Alison had been in and touched up my grey roots, and Mum had brought in my jeans, a leather jacket and my running shoes, so I was all dressed up with a place to go – home.

The nurses were all gathered around their station as I lifted myself out of the wheelchair and onto my crutches for the long walk home. 'Keep your bottom in,' the drill sergeant shouted as I tapped my crutches across the linoleum floor, my feet following the rhythm. My movements were mechanical but I was smiling. With each carefully taken step I felt more confident. I was leaving behind the high-dependency bay where I had spent the first two months of my rehabilitation. I passed the side ward where I had spent many a long afternoon gazing out across the garden, and kept walking with an unsteady but purposeful gait. As I walked more nurses followed behind me, I felt like Rocky leading a triumphant ringside circuit.

As I approached the doors that led off the ward I came to a halt. 'Hold your bottom up, you're sagging,' the drill sergeant prompted. But I could walk no further and came to a tearful halt slumping in a chair. Sara Short, who had trailed me all the way carrying my belongings in the hospital-issue plastic bag, helped me to sit down to catch my breath. I was overcome physically and emotionally. In all my determination to leave Osborn 4, I had not prepared myself for the sadness. Now as my therapists lined the corridor to say goodbye and other patients wheeled themselves towards me to shake my hand, I saw Becky, one of my favourite young nurses, crying as she stood at the side of the corridor waiting for me to walk past. Never again would she wipe my bottom, empty my catheter bag, spoon feed me Earl Grey tea, or make me laugh.

The finality hit me like a blow beneath the belt. I came to understand the impact these people had had on my life in the past six months. It's fair to say we had our share of ups and downs, mostly due to my impatience and what I perceived was their lack of empathy, but in all honesty these people had become my family. They had shared their knowledge with me and let me into their private lives, I felt like I was one of their friends. They had given me the medical knowledge and care to aid my successful recovery and allowed me to bend the rules along the way. I am not a sentimental person, but even I was overcome by the emotion. As I got back on my feet I could see my mum standing at the doors which led to the ordinary world. I staggered towards her for my last symbolic steps before crumpling into a waiting wheelchair. As I turned to wave my last farewell, I turned my head expecting to see the nurses giving me the rods. And I wouldn't have blamed them. But all I saw was a line of faces smiling through my sadness. True professionals to the end.

Thank You Isn't Enough ... You've all Saved What Could Have Been a Shit Life!

Posted on Facebook, Friday October 1 2010

I'm sat in my fab kitchen alone thinking about how people I know and don't know have given me the impetus to keep fighting. I really do believe that without your love and support, combined with my sheer bloody-mindedness, I wouldn't have come this far. From the bottom of my heart, thanks everyone and keep the encouragement coming, it gives me so much strength. Like Rocky on the steps in his famous film, I can hear the music now!

Chapter 38
OK Kids, Enough Already. Normality Returns

I KNEW THAT EIGHT months in hospital had made me institutionalised, but the actual shock of being back at home was greater than I had expected. Our family life was frenetic. After a couple of hours of being back in the hubbub of packed lunches, after-school clubs and sibling fights, I almost began to long for the boredom and relative quiet of the hospital ward.

Mark was still away on business so the in-laws, Ann and Kevin, were babysitting for both me and the children. They had put out the welcome home banners and balloons. As I unsteadily walked into the hall using my crutches, a homely smell wafted from the kitchen. Ann was roasting lamb for one of her famous dinners.

Looking forward, both sets of grandparents had said they wanted to start getting back to their own lives and could not continue the child-minding arrangement that had seen us through the hospital months. With my approval, Mark had hired our old babysitter Jessie for extra daily help. Monday to Friday she came in for three hours from 8 to 11 in the morning to get the children up and ready for school, walk Woody to school and cook dinner for me. Then in the afternoon she collected the children from school, packed their lunch boxes ready for the following morning, cooked their tea, and then took them to their various clubs. We also had a cleaner who came in for two hours a week before my stroke and while I was in hospital and she continued with this arrangement. For the first couple of months I relied heavily on this extra help. It worked well for both of us. Jessie was taking a year out after her A levels and needed the extra money and the children liked being with her. While I was still unsteady on my feet and could only walk a couple of metres on my crutches before I became tired, I needed someone around while Mark was in work.

The first night at home was strange. At bedtime Ann helped me upstairs to Harvey's bedroom. The bathroom was still a building site. I had trained myself not to drink anything after 7.30 so that I would not need to get up and use the toilet in the middle of the night and run the risk of falling over a piece of pipework. I slept like a board but at 2 a.m. and 6 a.m. I woke up. My body clock had been used to being woken up at these hours to be given drugs, and it took some time to readjust. Downstairs on the sofa bed the in-laws were also having a nervous, restless time, worried that I might fall during the night as I tried to get out of bed.

The following day Mark came home from Germany and we tried to pick up our lives as a family. Mark was a new man. After all the years of me moaning at him to pull his weight around the house, he was helping. He unpacked his bag and put his dirty washing in the laundry. He even did the ironing and filled the dishwasher. He was much more thoughtful and caring than the Mark I had left. 'At least there's been a positive by-product of the stroke,' I cheekily pointed out to him.

However the novelty of being a man about the house gradually wore off as my demands became more routine. Once I sat down I could not get up easily and would order Mark and the children to 'get the remote' or 'pass me my laptop'. My impatience also started to show. When I had been fit I did things myself, in my time. Depending on others always meant I had to wait and I hated waiting. This led to lots of friction and arguments. With me at home Mark also became more stressed, he was constantly worried that I would fall over or have an accident in the kitchen doing something I shouldn't. I have to say I never did, but it was something that always in the back of his mind. He always dreaded getting an emergency phone call in the middle of the day saying I had fallen or burnt myself on the cooker.

The children too found it strange having their mum back in their lives. Understandably they wanted to cling on to me but I felt like I was being smothered with their love and their hugs exhausted me. I also found myself getting wound up by the little things they did without even realising it. I had my favourite place to sit: on a stool at the corner of the breakfast bar. If one of the children had moved this stool there would be hell to pay, it was irrational I know but it took on a huge importance in my institutionalised mind. Gradually as I became more relaxed in my own surroundings, I made good use of the time on my own by practising my steps holding on to the island in the centre of our kitchen and walking around it in circuits. As I became more settled the children grew closer and took turns to sleep with me when Mark was away. This, in time, led to fights of another kind over who got the place in bed with me.

The mess was another thing that annoyed me when I first got home. One afternoon when I was on my own in between Jessie's shifts, I looked around the house at the papers piled high on table tops, toys littering the floor and thought 'what a tip'. Jessie had done a decent job of keeping all the surfaces clean and dust-free, but during the eight months I had been away no one had sorted through any paperwork. Enough was enough. I had to declutter. There were subscription renewal letters from Woody's Beavers group that hadn't been paid, bills that had been left for me to sort out, even Woody's Lego bricks, which had been in the corner of the lounge when I had the stroke, were still there gathering dust. In my absence Mark had been so concerned with getting on with life, he had had to allow some things to slip. Taking my time, I shuffled through piles of papers, sorting those that needed to be filed into one pile and putting the rest in another pile for Jessie to throw away. Papers and broken toys were all put out for the refuse. It was my way of putting my stamp back on our home.

It didn't take long before the children were back to their usual selves, shouting, fighting and throwing tantrums. Woody had always been the worst offender. Being the baby of the family he got the most attention; he was spoiled by everyone and disliked being told what to do more than his older brother and sister. His tantrums, although annoying, had never been an issue. When I had my full voice I could shout and put my foot down, but now it was physically impossible for me to raise my voice. If Mark was around he would step in but when I was on my own with him all I could do was reason with him quietly or leave him to come out of his sulk in his own time. Generally we muddled through and he knew how far he could push me but one night Woody threw such a tantrum that I had to call Alison to help me out. Woody was in the middle of playing a computer game when I told him it was time for bed. He saw red and started shouting and screaming. He stomped up to his room where he carried on throwing things around in temper. Mark was away and I was powerless to put an end to his bad behaviour. So I phoned Alison begging, 'Please, come and help me with Woody.' Hearing my desperation, Alison flew down to our house and in no time was putting Woody in his place. He stopped wrecking his bedroom and grudgingly picked up the toys he had thrown all over the floor. It was a lesson learnt. Don't push Mum too far, she has allies.

Chapter 39
I Will Run Again

ONCE HOME I COULD begin the gym routine that I had started to plan during my final weeks in hospital. I had set myself and Michael, my personal trainer, a target to get me running by Christmas. Initially Michael was dubious. I was in a wheelchair with weak, wobbly legs and just enough strength to support my own weight. I'm sure he must have secretly thought we would need a miracle to achieve my goal. If he did think this, he never said so. His positivity was just what I needed. After months of caution from the hospital therapists here was someone prepared to go at my pace.

Once I had left hospital I had just eight weeks of official therapy. The community physiotherapists visited the house once a week and set me exercises to walk up the first couple of stairs, which was pretty pathetic in my opinion, so I needed to set my own training programme and push myself harder.

Five times a week, the taxi came and collected me from home and took me on the ten-minute journey to the leisure club, where Michael met me and wheeled me through the concourse into the gym. The gym was huge, with bass-heavy dance music pumping in the background as the fit members pounded the treadmills and pumped iron. In my old life I had been a member of the leisure club for eight years and spent hours every week sweating it out on the cross-training machines and exercise bikes.

I felt the eyes of the other gym users watch me as Michael pushed me over to the leg press. They must have been questioning how someone who could not even walk properly was going to manage to lift weights. I should have been self-conscious, but I could not afford to be, I had to focus on the path ahead of me. To start with, Michael set me very basic exercises to strengthen my leg muscles. He helped me out of the chair on to the reclining squat machine. Lying on my back with my knees bent, feet pressing against the foot plate, I had to push my body weight away and straighten my knees. At first it was all I could do to manage two or three repetitions, but with every visit my resistance built up. Gradually I moved on to exercising using the lightest weight, struggling at first but slowly my muscles regained their strength and I moved up the weight scale.

For my upper body Michael helped me onto the chest press, where I used my stronger right arm to push the lightest of weight settings, gradually building up to more repetitions as I grew stronger. To build up my stamina Michael walked with me around the perimeter of the gym, steadying me with his arm. At first we managed just a few steps but over time I walked further. Like a child learning to ride a bike, my guiding hand would let go and I would step out confidently on my own. After six weeks of regular training I was able to ditch the wheelchair and walk into the gym on my crutches. As the other gym members got to know me they would offer to help me walk into the gym and this annoyed me. They were being kind, but I didn't want special treatment I thought to myself, 'You don't understand, I want to be normal like you, not dependent on you.' As I got stronger and fitter, Michael added more machines to my programme. Leg lifts, pectoral presses, five minutes on the cross trainer and exercise bikes. Even when I was a hundred per cent fit I had hated the treadmills, to me they were boring. I liked running in the open air. But Michael set me a walking programme starting at a 3km-an-hour pace – the aim was to build up to 4.8, which would be fast enough to attempt a run. At first I had trouble balancing on the treadmill and had to hold on to the hand rails for support, but as my confidence grew I was able to let go and speed up.

In addition to the daily gym routine I also started a weekly Pilates class with Anita in Dore village hall. Anita had tried to persuade me to go on many occasions in the past, but I had always declined. I had never been a fan of Pilates, all that concentration on stretching and breathing seemed boring to me. I liked my exercise hard and fast. But Anita convinced me now that it would be good for my balance. Twice a week we joined the other mums and retired ladies of the village to flex and bend and I have to admit it did help with my posture and balance. Anita also talked me into taking up singing lessons. Anita loves to sing, she is a member of the village choir, and was always the first one of us to burst into a tune on our girls' nights out. She reckoned that an hour a week with her teacher would help me control and strengthen my diaphragm and improve my speech. I tried it for a couple of months, but all that breathing in just left me light-headed, and singing the scales la-li-la-li-la fashion just made me feel silly, so I gave up after a couple of months. Anita also loaned me an old exercise bike, which I used religiously at home. There was only one problem: I needed help to get on and off.

At the end of November I said goodbye to my crutches. It was a happy day for me as I put them in the back of the wardrobe with the many pairs of shoes I had bought and only worn once. I would not be needing them again. I was confident of walking short distances on my own. However at this point it had become obvious that I was not going to achieve my ambitious goal of running by Christmas. I was disappointed but not distraught, as Michael explained that when I set my own goal I had massively underestimated the time that learning to pick up my knees and run would take. Walking, although hard, required fewer muscles to move one foot in front of the other with legs almost straight. On the positive side I had just completed my first continuous one kilometre on the cross trainer and I was up to half a kilometre on the treadmill, both of which left me absolutely knackered. To run I had to learn to perfect the leg movement of the cross trainer but without holding on to the handles. I wasn't quite there yet, but Michael was confident that if I kept up the hard work I would be running by February.

I decided I would mark the anniversary of my stroke on February 6 with a charity run. I posted a message on Facebook saying that I'd run through my local Eccleshall Wood and all my friends and fellow runners were welcome to join me. Three months – no pressure.

Chapter 40
A Weekend Away With the Girls

I HAD BEEN HOME just three days when I packed my bag for my first weekend away with the girls. Every September Anita and I and a group of other mums would leave our families for an all-girls weekend break. The previous couple of years we had gone to Spain and memories of these trips had kept me going through the dark times in hospital. This year was to be different.

After everything that we had been through as friends, Anita didn't have the heart to organise a holiday in Spain as it was unlikely I could go with them. Ever thoughtful, she suggested that we could do something closer to home. In the weeks before I had left hospital, I had something to look forward to as Anita talked of possible places we could visit. With my recovery taking great leaps, Anita left it until the last minute to book and presented me with a fait accompli – an overnight trip to Champneys Springs, a luxury spa resort in Leicestershire, for Saturday October 2. A group of six would be going. I was still mostly using the wheelchair to get around at this point, so she booked Alison and me into a twin room with wheelchair access.

On the morning of our departure, Anita collected us in the back of her Mercedes van for the ninety-minute drive to the spa. It felt good to be back in the company of all my friends, which had been one of the things I had missed most when I was in hospital and was restricted to two visitors at a time. When we arrived, we offloaded our bags and started planning our fitness classes. There was a programme of aerobics, tai chi, legs, bums and tums, and meditation sessions. The choice of massage and pampering treatments seemed endless, with chocolate wraps and lime and ginger salt glows, which sounded like a restaurant menu. Anita and some of the other mums took full advantage of the pampering on offer. Alison, who was my room mate for the night, used me as an excuse to avoid anything that required too much exertion. We both booked ourselves a facial massage for later in the afternoon and went off to find a lounger at the poolside. We were given a private changing area with disabled access and Alison helped me to change into my swimming costume. Getting into the pool took some time. The side of the pool was wet and slippery and I was conscious that I didn't want to fall and embarrass myself in front of the other hotel guests, so with Alison by my side to steady me I carefully picked my way to the water's edge and got in.

Once in the pool I had to use a child's life ring to help me support my head. I had been swimming a couple of times with my physiotherapists in Osborn 4 and they had helped support my body weight but when I went on my own with Mark I almost drowned. I just did not have the strength in my body to keep me afloat. 'I feel daft wearing this,' I said self-consciously to Alison, who reminded me I shouldn't care what other people thought. After a while I got over my embarrassment and just enjoyed the time for what it was, a relaxing, carefree weekend.

We spent the entire afternoon chilling around the pool until I turned to Alison and said, 'Is it wine time

245

yet?'

'I thought you would never ask,' she replied. For her, it was another sign that I was getting back to my old self. The pair of us went to our rooms and cracked open a bottle of Cava to celebrate.

But before we could get to our room, we had the obstacle of getting through the double doors. Anita had booked a room with disabled access, but this room was in a different wing of the building from the other girls, and to get to it we had to negotiate a steep incline and two sets of double doors. We laughed as Alison turned into a contortionist, trying to hold onto my chair to stop it rolling downhill, while wedging the door open with her legs. I tried to help by holding the door as much as I could but it was difficult and a reminder that even places with disabled access aren't always easy to use.

When the time came for Alison to go and have her facial, she asked Anita if she would collect me after my treatment and bring me back to the room. 'Of course,' said Anita, who was happy to be using her nurturing and maternal skills.

After my massage, there was no one there to meet me. I waited and waited. No Anita. After half an hour the therapist rang our room and Alison answered. Anita had completely forgotten she was supposed to collect me, so the therapist kindly took me back. Once I was safely back in the room, Alison couldn't resist winding up Anita, who was actually drinking gin and tonic in the bar with the other girls. Alison called and asked if I was with her, knowing that I was not. When Anita hesitated, Alison said, 'I hope you haven't left her behind. You know how upset she will be.' Anita was distraught. Then Alison pretended that I had just been brought back to the room and was in tears. 'Can you hear how upset she is?' she asked down the phone. I played along, putting on my best donkey voice to sound like I was crying. Anita was so embarrassed and unusually lost for words. It was a cruel joke for Alison to play on her, but it made us laugh all weekend.

The rest of the break was just as much fun. For me it was a great opportunity to reconnect with all the friends who had stayed by my side through the difficult times. They had laughed with me when I was a dribbling, drooling mess and now we could all laugh together like old times. My disability was not an issue, no one treated me any differently, even though I lagged behind. The old Kate would have been the last one to go to bed, but that night I was the first to leave the bar and ask Alison to take me back to my room. I told her to go back to join the rest of the girls while I went to sleep, I was exhausted but happy.

Inspired by our weekend away, I went on to organise many other get-togethers. I started back to book club and immersed myself in a world of fiction and fantasy. All the time I had been in hospital, the book club had suffered, particularly in the early days when my friends had found it difficult to concentrate their minds on the escapism that reading could bring. Unless the books were other memoirs of overcoming severe illness, they could not find the enthusiasm to discuss them. Now we were back in action and I chose a real-life memoir *Deceived* by Sarah Smith. I was engrossed in the story of how this young student had been manipulated for ten years by a conman who made her think he was an MI5 agent and she was escaping from the IRA.

With Jaqui, Alison and Anita's help I also organised a surprise party for Mark's forty-fourth birthday the weekend after my spa break. For eight months I had been hogging the limelight and I wanted to make Mark feel special. I managed to keep it a secret and arranged for a group of friends to meet at Jaqui's house, where we had decorated the room with Chinese lanterns and birthday banners. Mark thought we were going to the local pub when the taxi came to pick us up, but instead we made the trip to Jaqui's house where all our friends were waiting. The look on Mark's face as he saw all his friends and a banquet of Chinese food laid out for him was priceless. Even though I was still weak and unable to eat the rich takeaway food, I was happy to see him relaxed and having fun.

Chapter 41
Till Death Us Do Part

BEING BACK HOME WITH Mark made me rethink our whole relationship. While I had been insecure and scared that he might leave me for a newer model he could have a decent conversation with– or even a dumb blonde with a healthy sexual appetite, the time in hospital made me realise his love for me was unconditional. Throughout my recovery he had selflessly held the family together and had even given me the spirit to fight on with his sometimes insensitive comments. He had stood by the vows for richer or poorer, in sickness and in health, and I wanted to give something back – so I proposed.

The idea came to me back on Osborn 4 while I was watching *This Morning* where a woman who had renewed her vows after surviving a life-threatening illness was being interviewed. When I saw Mark later that night I asked, 'Do you fancy getting married again?' His response was underwhelming. He looked at me as if I was pulling his leg. It was hardly the grand romantic gesture of our original wedding when he had flown halfway round the world to win back my love. We were sitting in the middle of a hospital ward surrounded by brain-injured patients, but I wasn't put off. 'I mean it,' I said. 'Let's renew our vows.' With some hesitation, he agreed.

He later admitted that he thought it was a load of 'old mumbo' and I was making it up. Once he had given it some thought, though, he appreciated the reasons we had to reconfirm the promises we had made in 1998, and that it would be a good excuse to throw a big celebration party. I had started to make the arrangements from hospital. I had emailed the priest at Dore church, who came to see me in hospital, and we had set the date for Sunday May 15 – our thirteenth wedding anniversary. Unlucky, some might say.

I also started shopping online for something to wear. I found just what I was looking for at Coast, a simple black and white, off-the-shoulder dress. I rang the branch at Meadowhall Shopping Centre to ask if they had it in my size. But before I could get the words out, the shop assistant on the other end had hung up thinking I was a hoax caller. This really knocked my confidence and has since led me to start all phone calls with a need to explain my poor speech. I now start every phone call with 'Don't hang up. I'm not a hoax, I've had a stroke.' It made me realise how prejudiced and intolerant of disabilities some people can be. The next day Alison took me to the shop in person and gave the shop assistant a piece of her mind. We found the dress in a size 10 and took it home to try on. As Alison zipped me up, I lost my balance and fell over, unable to save myself. Luckily I had a soft landing when the sofa broke my fall. Alison could hardly lift me back on my feet, she was laughing so much.

At home I started working on the finer details of wedding planning, booking the local rugby club for the reception and organising caterers. I wanted this to be a celebration of life as well as love witnessed by the friends who had helped us get back to normal life. I sent out a Facebook invitation to all my friends and family.

'Some of you may know it's our wedding anniversary and what better way to celebrate? All welcome. Pressies not necessary, we want a fab holiday instead to America as a family! Kids welcome and nurses! RSVP ME. Is anyone a veggie? I need RSVPs because we are not sending formal invites, but need to know for catering!

Our first wedding had been fun. We had held it at Whitely Hall, a beautiful sixteenth-century mansion house hotel in south Yorkshire. After the reception, the boys from the rugby club played cricket on the lawn in the blazing sun. The party in the evening was a seventies-themed disco, a sea of purple crushed velvet, long wigs and flowing tunics. I remember Mark's parents refused to leave before the bride, so at 4 a.m. they were still partying!

Instead of a honeymoon this time, I had planned a two-week holiday to Disney World in Florida. Again I had started organising the trip while I was in hospital. Donna, my old school friend, worked at a travel agent's and she helped me with a good deal on flights and renting a villa. The doctors had finally given me clearance to fly and the Stroke Association had helped me find travel insurance which didn't cost the earth.

Making grand public gestures of our commitment was one thing, but for months after I returned home I had had problems with the physical side of our relationship. Psychologically I had issues, I couldn't handle intimacy. For so long my body had been the public property of the doctors and nurses, who probed and prodded all my private nooks and crannies. Once I was home I could say, 'Sod off, it's my body, I've had enough invasion.' It took some time, but gradually Mark and I were able to rekindle our physical relationship with an emotional intensity that I never thought was possible.

Our bedroom was also the scene of many funnier episodes. I kept a walking frame by the side of the bed in case I needed to go to the toilet during the night. I would get out of bed, waking Mark up as I did, and shuffle to the bathroom. At these times Mark reckoned I hit every piece of furniture with the frame on purpose, just to make sure he was awake and knew I was on the move. The truth of the matter was that, in the darkness, it was difficult to manoeuvre and there were occasions when I didn't make it to the bathroom but ended up in a heap on the floor, laughing and waiting for Mark to pick me up.

Chapter 42
Danger Lurks in Turkey and Meatballs

HAVING FOUGHT SO HARD to get out of hospital, imagine how pissed off I was when I ended up back in A&E just a few weeks later, thanks to a turkey curry. My gullet had always been narrower than most people's. I remember as a child my parents would always tell me to chew my food as it would get stuck in my food pipe, but now that I had less muscle function, I had to take even more care.

For the first few weeks after leaving hospital I had been pureeing my food then, as I felt stronger, I had moved on to solids. One of the long-term effects of the stroke was to leave me with weak muscles in my oesophagus. I have adopted new rules for eating. I have to take small bites and concentrate on chewing each mouthful well. Sometimes I have to use my finger to move the food around my mouth as my tongue muscles are not strong enough. When I swallow, I always have to tuck my chin in to close my windpipe and open my oesophagus to avoid choking. Occasionally, if I feel the food going down the wrong way I have a toothbrush on hand and tickle the back of my throat, as I was shown by the ward manager on Osborn 4. This causes an involuntarily cough to push the offending particle back up because I cannot cough at will. If I follow these rules

I can avoid any dramas and while it may sound like an extremely convoluted way to eat for normal people, it was important to me. My social life revolved around eating and drinking, whether it was my Earl Grey tea with Jaqui and Anita after our Saturday morning runs, or the Friday nights at our local curry house. This was one of the reasons I insisted on having the PEG removed.

Yet even with all these measures in place I managed to choke on a turkey curry. I was at home with Mark and the children one evening when it happened. I'm not sure how, as I was following all the precautions, but the turkey became lodged halfway down my food pipe and refused to move. I tried washing it down with coke, but it would not shift. I could feel it stuck in my neck, going nowhere. It was causing a burning pain in my chest, so there was no other way round it, I would have to go back to Accident & Emergency. Mark called our babysitter to sit with the children and drove me to the casualty department at our nearest hospital, Sheffield Hallam. From there I was transferred to the Ear, Nose and Throat department, where further investigation revealed that the turkey was too low for them to see it with their regular equipment. I was admitted to an overnight ward as plans were made for me to have an endoscopy the following day. 'No way,' I thought as I was given a bed on the gastro ward for the night and Mark went back home. I had spent enough time in hospital to last me a lifetime, there was no way I was going to waste another night lying awake on an NHS bed if it wasn't absolutely necessary.

When the doctor came round with the results of my X-rays I decided I was getting out. He explained that the meat had moved down and was not near my windpipe but they would need to take me into surgery the

254

following morning and push a telescopic tube down inside me to dislodge the meat. I decided there and then that if the obstruction was not in danger of blocking my windpipe I was safe and in time it would slide down. So I wanted out. After the doctor left, I played hell with the nurses, demanding they let me go home. When they refused I pulled out the cannula, which had already been inserted in the back of my hand in preparation for the morning's pre-surgery blood test and discharged myself. I called Mark to come and collect me and I was gone. I slept that night with a small amount of discomfort from the lodged meat but, like I thought, it gradually slipped into my stomach as I moved around the next morning.

With this drama over, I quickly found my way back into a social routine with my friends. Anita and Alison would pop in for coffee, I treated myself to tea and cake in the Esporta coffee shop after a particularly hard gym session, and we also resumed our Friday night pub routine. Friday night was scouts and guides night for India, Harvey and Alison's daughters. So we dropped the children off in the village hall at 6.30 p.m. then retreated to the village pub with Woody and Nicole for a couple of hours until it was time to collect them. One thing I soon discovered was my tolerance to alcohol had changed. Before my stroke I happily drank one or two glasses of red wine or a couple of gin and tonics, now I found that most alcohol tasted foul. It was harsh on my delicate throat so on these occasions I would just have a soft drink like the children, or if I really wanted to push the boat out I ordered vodka with lots of coke, which was the one drink I could stomach. The important thing for me was feeling part of the community again, sitting in the pub, talking to friends and villagers about the routine of life, not just my stroke. As we re-established our Friday nights out, people started seeing through the slow, deliberate speech and the ungainly walking which were reminders of the stroke, to recognise the old Kate.

Not everyone was so kind and accepting. I remember one afternoon I had been to have my hair done in Alison's salon. It was a Saturday afternoon and I was the last customer. When Alison closed up the shop we went to the pub on the corner for a quick one before going home. I had left Alison to lock up and gone on ahead to order our drinks. The pub was screening a big match and it was unusually busy, full of students and rugby fans. As I walked into the pub slowly and unsteadily, without my crutches for support, I could see the drinkers sitting in the window seats staring out at me. I felt as though they were looking at me and judging, thinking I was pissed. It was a sharp reminder of how we humans are quick to judge others who do not conform to our idea of 'normal'. I'm sure when I was a student I would have had the same reaction, but now I had learned the hard way that you should not judge a book by its cover, and just because someone is staggering into the pub doesn't mean they have had a few too many. A year ago, maybe, but not now.

On another night out with Mark and Alison I found myself the centre of attention at our Indian restaurant. The entire day had been a drama. It was the day before Woody's seventh birthday and I was organising his party for the next day. During dinner I choked on a meatball. I knew straight away as soon as it left my mouth that it was too big and was going to cause me grief. Like the turkey, it jammed itself halfway down my oesophagus, causing a pain that felt as if I was being stabbed in the back. I tried drinking Coke to wash it down, but it was going nowhere. In desperation I turned to the superior medical knowledge of Google for some suggestions on how to cure a trapped meatball. I tried drinking water bending over. I even drank a raw egg, but it would not shift. I could feel it in my throat. Being a Friday night I didn't fancy my chances with all the drunks at A&E so I waited and spent an uncomfortable night in bed, the pain never letting up. The following morning it had not moved, so visited the A&E department. Again the doctors wanted to keep me in until Monday morning when the consultant was on duty and would be able to perform the endoscopy to push the meat into my stomach. I pleaded with them to let me go sooner. The next day was Woody's birthday party and Mark was going to South Africa on business. 'I have to go home tonight,' I begged. Thankfully the consultant was called in and carried out the procedure under local anaesthetic. My guess is that they were short on beds for the weekend, but I was delighted. By 10 p.m. that night I was sitting at my local curry house with Mark, Alison and her husband, eating poppadums and drinking vodka and Coke waiting for my prawn starter. I had not eaten for more than twenty-four hours and I was starving.

Suddenly I felt a searing pain in my stomach and I slumped forward in my chair. Panicking Mark lifted me from the table and carried me out to the entrance, laying me out on the cold stone floor while the waiter called for an ambulance. The other diners in the restaurant must have thought I had passed out through too much drink.

'Don't leave me Kate. I couldn't live without you,' I heard him whimper above all the commotion. My head felt light. Alison held my hand in hers and asked me to squeeze. I did. 'Cancel the ambulance, Mark, she's only fainted,' Alison shouted across the restaurant. As I came round, I noticed that my new white blouse was covered in sauce. 'Do you think this stain will come out?' I asked Alison as Mark looked at me, his face a mixture

257

of relief and disbelief. With hindsight, drinking vodka on an empty stomach was not the wisest move.

Chapter 43
Charity Begins at Home

WINSTON CHURCHILL WAS QUOTED as saying 'Success is not final, failure is not fatal. It's the courage to continue that counts.' I quite agree with the great man. We all have a choice whether we want to fight on to achieve our goals or roll over and admit defeat for fear of never reaching them. For me it was a no-brainer. When it was clear I had survived the stroke, I had no choice but to get better and get back to my normal life, even if my friends and family had shielded me from the negativity of the medics who were sceptical about a fast and full recovery. In my mind being disabled was a transient stage in my life. Once I was out of the ICU and on the road to recovery I never once thought I wouldn't be the Kate I once was, even if everyone else had their doubts.

When I decided to set up a charity Fighting Strokes Young and Locked-In Syndrome, Churchill's quote became my mission statement. Before February 6 2010, I had never heard of locked-in syndrome and thought that strokes were something that happened to old people. But as I began to reconnect with the world via Facebook, I soon discovered that I was not alone in my locked-in state. It seemed that I was one of the lucky ones. I had been locked in for only eight weeks before I started to show flickers of movement. I say only, but many of the people who remained locked-in died.

On the internet I started reading up on well-known cases from across the world. Not just those of famous people like Jean-Dominique Bauby, the author of The *Diving Bell and the Butterfly* or the American Julia Tavalaro, who was thirty-two when she suffered two strokes and spent six years in a vegetative state before anyone realised she was alive inside. There were more positive stories too like Graham Miles, an Englishman from Sussex who was forty-nine when he suffered his brain stem stroke and started walking twenty years later. I also took inspiration from the true stories of survivors of other near-death illnesses. The one that moved me the most was Lance Armstrong's book *It's Not About The Bike: My Journey Back to Life*. In his fight to recover from cancer and win the world's most famous and gruelling bike race the Tour de France plus set up a cancer foundation and benefit bike ride, I saw some of my own hurdles. I could understand his commitment to get better and his never-ending drive despite all the odds, it made me feel I had more to offer others.

When a friend helped me to set up my Beating Locked-in Syndrome page on Facebook I was overwhelmed by the response. Within the first few weeks I gathered 500 friends, which grew to 1,000 over time. Not only were my friends and family reading my thoughts but there were strangers from as far away as New York and Spain who found inspiration in my story.

One man in New York told me about his friend Sheila Keegan Uhl, who suffered a similar stroke on Boxing Day. He wrote:

'We have all been inspired by your story and comforted by the knowledge that there is real hope. I'm sure that any words of advice and encouragement you can give to Sheila and her family would provide a huge boost as she makes progress each and every day in this uphill battle. Thank you for sharing your positive energy with us.'

The mother of a young man in America also contacted me after finding my story on the internet. She wrote:

'Want to let you know you have been an inspiration to our family. Our son, Stephen, had a catastrophic brain stem stroke on October 15. His prognosis was very poor, 'Locked-in Syndrome' at the best. We began researching LIS and found your site and read your story to Steve. Shortly after, he began responding and waking up. He is in a rehabilitation facility and engaged in speech/swallowing, physical and occupational therapies, moving all limbs now and talking (no voice, due to trachi/so we are struggling to read his lips). He is still on a ventilator. There is a long, hard road ahead, but Steve is very committed to his recovery. Thank you and keep running!'

In September 2010, a young man called Gary Atkinson also suffered a brain-stem stroke which left him with Locked-In Syndrome. His situation was almost identical to mine. His young daughter Chloe had been following my Facebook page and out of the blue I had an email from his wife Deborah. She explained Gary's situation and asked if I would be willing to go and visit her husband fifty miles away in Bury, Lancashire.

Her email read:

'I have followed your story with great interest since finding out about your unbelievable and remarkable strength in recovering from a brain-stem stroke and locked-in syndrome. Just like your husband and you, we were given very negative news of doom and gloom about Gary's future. Being a very positive person myself and after reading of how you fought through

261

locked-in syndrome and came out of it, I was not about to give in for Gary I have a lot to prove and I know Gary has inner strength that he will draw on. I want to prove to medics that why not – if someone else has come through this then why can't Gary? At present Gary is six months in to his illness in a rehabilitation unit in Bury, where he is receiving daily therapy including physiotherapy, speech, language therapy, psychology and occupational therapy as well as general nursing care. I just wondered what therapy you were receiving at this stage in your recovery. I don't wish you to be reminded of the calendar of events and emotions that you went through but your symptoms and diagnosis were like a mirror image of Gary's and I know that it would help me to encourage Gary to keep up the fight. At present Gary keeps suffering with little niggling infections which seem to knock us back a little when things are progressing well. I would love to try and help in some way to support your fight to highlight locked-in syndrome.'

To these people I replied as best I could, sharing my experience and telling them to help their loved ones to set and achieve goals, no matter how small or insignificant. Around this time I also had an email from Hazel Cushion, the managing director of book publisher Accent Press who had read how I was writing a book and offered me a book deal. Another of my hospital goals was being realised, all those notes I had scribbled down in my long and lonely hours in Osborn 4 would now be made into a book.

Through Facebook I also met another mother from the Midlands. Sue was married with a thirteen-year-old son and a grown-up son. She had suffered a stroke that summer and lost her movement. Like me she was determined that she would walk again and pushed for therapy to help her walk up stairs. She also offered to support my charity and join the fight for others.

As my story spread through the online stroke community I also found myself at the centre of media attention. I became a regular contributor to online forums where carers of stroke patients discussed their positive steps and shared their frustrations. I was invited to speak on a radio debate on the subject of whether families should be given the right to switch off their next of kin's life support without fear of being prosecuted by police. Naturally my argument was no. My story was also spotted by a journalist from the *Daily Mirror* who drove more than 200 miles to interview me. The interview appeared in the centre pages on Friday November 5. I was gobsmacked: Kate Allatt, centrefold. Thank God it wasn't page three. When Dave read the article he burst into tears. Seeing my story in print brought back the hardest time of his life, there were still so many raw emotions.

I wasn't prepared for the reaction that followed. TV, radio and women's magazines all wanted my story. However I didn't feel ready for my big primetime TV debut yet as my speech was still weak. I did, however, agree to an interview on my local BBC Radio Sheffield as I had been on their afternoon show with presenter Rony Robinson just three days before the stroke happened. I sat in the studio waiting to go on air as Rony played the Bee Gees hit 'Staying Alive', appropriate choice of music, I thought. Then he introduced me by playing the recording I made in the studio on February 3. Listeners heard a chirpy, excited young Kate talking about plans to climb Mount Kilimanjaro for the local children's hospice. Then he switched on the microphone and his listeners heard my stroke voice as I relived what happened next. In a matter-of-fact way I described the day of the stroke, my feelings of being buried alive and wanting to die, the anger at being written off and the inspiration my children, family and friends gave me to walk and talk again. I thanked the people of Dore for the community spirit that helped me and my family pull through the dark times. And finally I explained my ambition to run again on February 6, the anniversary of my stroke, and my new goal to set up a charity to help other young stroke survivors. After the interview Rony opened up the telephone line to listeners for their comments and was amazed by the reaction. He said that in his twenty-six years as a broadcaster he had never experienced a reaction like it. One man texted in and said, 'I had to stop my car to wipe away the tears for that lovely Kate who showed so much bravery and courage.' Another called to say he was also in tears to hear my story. A woman who was on her way to church to arrange her mother's funeral when she heard my story and said it put everything into perspective; she thanked me for my inspiration. Another said she had a friend in Grantham who had also suffered a major stroke and hearing my words gave her hope for her friend. The calls kept coming in: each one more emotional than the last. I might sound hard but I felt detached about hearing complete strangers crying over me. It was as if the Kate they were hearing about was a different person, from another period in time.

I could not understand what the fuss was about, it was just my life and I had got over it. I was moving on. However this interest in my life made me realise just how vital my charity could be in giving young people with strokes the support and encouragement they needed on the long road to recovery. The Stroke Association estimate that of 150,000 people in the UK who have a stroke each year only 10,000 are under retirement age, and an even smaller percentage are forty or under, so this would be the area my charity would focus on.

Campaigning was another area in which I wanted my charity to take a lead. One of the first cases I was happy to get involved in was the case of Michelle Wheatley, a young mother-of-two from Stockport, Greater Manchester. Michelle's parents, Linda and Frank, had contacted me for support in their fight to get Michelle intensive therapy at a private clinic. Michelle was just twenty-seven when she became locked in. For two years she had been living in a residential care home with blinking her only means of communication while her partner was left to look after their two young children. Her family had raised £17,000 to help her and in a last-ditch attempt wanted their NHS Trust to spend £42,000 on a twelve-week intensive therapy programme at a private clinic. The health board was refusing, claiming it would be no better than her present therapy. They turned to me as an example of how the right therapy could achieve the results they needed. Michelle's story touched me and I agreed to visit her to give her some words of inspiration.

Alison came with me and together we made the forty-mile trip to Stockport to meet Michelle and her family. Secretly Alison was worried how I would react when I saw Michelle, knowing that it could have been me in that care home. I didn't give it a second thought. What I saw in Michelle was a fighter. She had a system of communicating where she looked up for yes and down for no, which made it difficult to make eye contact. I thought how my expressive eyes had spoken much more than the words on my chart. Using a communication board, I asked Michelle what she liked to do. 'SHOPPING' she blinked as her parents showed me a pair of black high heels she had bought on one of her recent day trips to the shops.

I explained to Michelle and her family how she needed to set herself small, but achievable goals. 'Imagine yourself standing up and walking in your new shoes,' I suggested. Michelle's eyes lit up. I could tell that locked inside Michelle's body was a kindred spirit. She had fight and spark and that, with the right therapy, could be channelled into positive recovery. I happily supported Michelle's fight and, three days after my visit, Michelle's parents told me they had won their case. Michelle was getting a second bite of the cherry. As I explained to Michelle's parents, I truly believe in mind over matter. If your mind is cognitive you can do all sorts. The power of the brain is massively underestimated.

With the mission and aims of my charity clear, I needed an identity. An ex-work colleague and graphic designer agreed to come up with a logo which combined the three important elements representing my fight back to health and fitness. The eye with the lock in the centre symbolised being locked in and my only means of communication – blinking, while the iconic image of Rocky with his fist in the air symbolised my ongoing inspiration. Rocky was the underdog who beat the odds and won. My charity would fight for those medical underdogs who were given no hope. With that in mind I sat down and penned a letter to my *Rocky* hero, Sylvester Stallone, asking if he would be a patron of my charity. I await his reply.

Chapter 44
'All We Want for Christmas is our Mum'

I DON'T NORMALLY DO public displays of emotion, among my friends I'm the hard-nosed one. So why was it that on Christmas Day I kept crying all day? Being in the heart of my family, watching the children get more and more excited the closer we got to Christmas Eve, made me appreciate how different it could all have been.

The week before Christmas I was invited back to Osborn 4 for the ward's Christmas party. The nurses and patients who remembered me were astonished by how well I looked and how much I had progressed. I was less reliant on my crutches to walk even though I kept them for support. I told the staff about my plans to make my first run on the anniversary of my stroke and several of the nurses signed up to join me.

Christmas Eve was the only time we ever went to church, for the Dore candlelit Christmas carol service. It was a ritual in the village which all my friends and their children and even their husbands would join in. It was one of the highlights of the Dore community calendar. However the children had warned me that I was not allowed to sing. Considering I had been having singing lessons for the past two months, I thought this was a bit

267

harsh. But then I remembered the embarrassment I had caused during India's school concert with my donkey-like laugh and agreed it was probably sensible to keep my mouth shut. It was strange sitting in the church and not joining in with my favourite carol 'Good King Wenceslas'. So I did the next best thing and sneezed. It started as a tickle in the back of my nose and erupted as a force-ten explosion during the quietest point of the service in the middle of the vicar's address. How embarrassing.

As the service ended I found myself the centre of attention once again. Whether it was the sneeze or the stroke, I can't be sure, but people who I had not seen since the last Christmas Eve came up to wish me well. It felt so good to be out doing normal things.

After the service we did the Christian thing and went to the village pub for a pre-Christmas drink before going home to get ready for Father Christmas. India and Harvey did not actually believe in Santa but they humoured me for Woody's sake as we put out a bucket of water and a carrot in the garden for Rudolph and a mince pie and glass of Baileys for Santa before going off to bed.

Christmas Day was surprisingly emotional. I found myself bursting into tears for the least thing. Mark and I had decided that we would make it the best Christmas ever. The children had had a rubbish ten months and we agreed there was to be no limit to the budget. We would go overboard and give them everything they had put on their Santa list, which was surprisingly modest for once. I had been shopping online: there were designer clothes and trainers for India, a cricket set and Manchester United soccer strip for Harvey and a scooter for Woody.

At 7 a.m. on Christmas Day a trio of excited faces peeped around our bedroom door dragging their stockings behind them. As they tore open the wrapping from their presents they each said how they wished they could have wrapped themselves up and given themselves to me. I cried. India took me to one side and confessed, 'Mum, I know about Father Christmas and I'm very grateful for everything he brought me. But I'm just glad you're here.' Again, I blubbed like a baby.

To complete the Christmas card picture of the perfect family, Mark lit the fire and as the snow in the garden thawed, we sat around the fire playing games and cuddling together in the heat of the flames.

Lunchtime brought more emotions. Roast dinner was my favourite meal, the first meal I ate properly after my PEG came out, and Christmas dinner was the best of all. But after the turkey choking incident I was extra careful to tilt my head forward and eat slowly without speaking, which was quite a challenge.

While Christmas Day was a time for us to be close together as a family, relaxing and enjoying one another's company, Boxing Day was open house. All day and well into the night friends and neighbours called in to share a drink and a chat. On both Christmas and Boxing Day I found myself tiring quickly and went to bed far earlier than was civilised for a party girl, but I just didn't have the stamina to party like the old Kate.

I had some good news myself over Christmas. On Thursday December 30 I went back to Northern General Hospital to see my consultant neurologist Ming the Merciless for the first check-up since leaving hospital. I walked into the consultation room unaided and sat before his desk. He was amazed at what he saw.

'You are a miracle! You must have had divine intervention,' he said. I soon set him straight.

'It's called bloody hard work,' I told him. It annoyed

me that he was devaluing all the effort I had put in to reach the point I had. He did, however, give me a piece of good news – I was fit to drive. I could have kissed him. Ever since I had found out that Mark had sold my car when I was in the ICU I had set my sights on a new car – a red Mini convertible. I had been lucky that Mark, despite all his efficiency, had forgotten to send my driving licence back to the DVLA. My consultant explained that he used to be a driving instructor and he was happy to fill in the medical form that declared me fit to drive. A couple of weeks later Mark, true to his word, surprised me with a late Christmas present: a red Mini convertible. I called it Rocky, after my inspirational movie hero. With my new wheels I had even greater independence, I could walk from the house to the car and drive wherever I wanted to go. No longer did I need to rely on taxis to take me to and from the gym. If I wanted to meet a friend for coffee in town, I could get in the car and go. I had a disabled badge, so I could park close to wherever I needed to go. I took a couple of weeks to master clutch control again, kangaroo jumps becoming my speciality.

Compared to Christmas, New Year's Eve 2010 was a low-key affair. Alison and her husband Chris came around with their kids. Alison and I spent most of the evening in the kitchen on our own, neither of us had any inclination to celebrate auld acquaintances and all that rubbish. Alison was missing her dad and I could not see the point in making any grand plans. I had done that last year and look where it had got me. I managed to stay up till midnight, the latest since I had been out of hospital, and toasted in a brighter 2011 before retiring to bed.

That night I posted on Facebook: 'So the end of 2010, I can't say I'm sad about it! It's been a year like no other. But I'm still here and however tired this little fighter Rocky is, I will continue to keep fighting to be back like I was, for all young people with strokes and particularly locked-in syndrome. Thank you for following; it gives me so much strength to keep fighting it every day. The glass is NOT half empty, but half full!'

Chapter 45
Running Is My Freedom

SUNDAY FEBRUARY 6 2011 was the day when I could close this chapter of my life and move on.

It was a year to the day since my stroke and the day when I promised myself and everyone else that I would run again. Symbolically it was a big step in my recovery. For my friends and family it was a celebration of my survival but for me it was more a statement: I had said I would run again and I would.

I had posted an invitation to the event on my Facebook page, starting at my house at noon. Anita had planned a couple of walking and running routes from 1km to 5km and would lead the run, all my friends and family and villagers were welcome to take part.

In the weeks leading up to the anniversary, I had managed to run up to twenty metres at a time with my personal trainer by my side. As friends started to gather at my house that Sunday morning, the butterflies arrived in my stomach. My serious running friends and Mark's biking friends turned up in their outdoor gear, school mums and their children were there in their leggings and trainers and the grandparents and older members of the church were ready in their walking boots. One of the young doctors who had last seen me when she took care of me in the ICU all those months earlier was there to take part and was astounded by my progress. Even Alison, who constantly reminded me, 'I don't do running,' was kitted out in her trainers, her view on this momentous occasion was that if I could do it she could not refuse. There was also a camera crew from our local TV news filming for that evening's news bulletin, so there was no pressure.

As I tied the laces on my running shoes, a task which just six months ago had taken me five hours to complete, I started to panic. What if I couldn't do it? What if I failed and embarrassed myself? The truth was that no one on the run would have cared, but I had my pride. My trainer was convinced I could do it. Like an elite athlete he took me to one side and gave me a pep talk and strapped my weak left calf with a special tape, which is used by the likes of David Beckham, Lance Armstrong and Andy Murray to enhance their performance. In my case it was to support my weaker muscles and allow them better movement.

At 12 noon the crowds of people who had gathered in the house and spilled out into the garden walked to the start of the run. Just as I was getting into my personal trainer's car to be chauffeured to the starting point I heard someone call my name. Sue, the fellow mum and stroke survivor who I had only met via Facebook, together with her thirteen-year-old son and husband, had made the two-hour journey from her home to cheer me on. In all more than 150 people gathered at the starting line including Michelle Wheatley's parents who were hoping to take home inspiration for their daughter. It made me realise that this event was not just important to me.

All eyes were on me. As I stepped out of the car and onto the muddy track to take my position at the head of the pack, I was overwhelmed. Holding onto my trainer for support, I steadied myself and inhaled deeply. Then I was off. Running free. One metre, two metres, ten metres and counting. At fifteen metres I stopped to catch my breath, holding on to my trainer for support, I could see tears of joy on the faces of my friends. Even the TV reporter, whom I had only met an hour ago, was choking back her emotions. I had been determined to achieve my own personal goal, but now I could see just how much my recovery meant to others. My fight had left a lasting imprint on my close family, but I had also touched the lives of others like Sue and the Wheatleys. It inspired me to fight on for others who didn't have my drive. I couldn't contain my emotions any longer, the 'Iron Lady' cracked and broke down in tears, cameras recording my moment of achievement.

'Come on, you can do another five metres,' my trainer pushed. I breathed deeply, wiped the tears from my face, held tightly onto Alison's waist for support and carried on. The mud squelched under my new running shoes as I counted down the distance, laughing through the tears. At twenty metres I called it a day and shouted, 'I think I deserve a drink. Who's coming to the pub with me?'

I stood at the bar of our village pub, pouring celebration glasses of pink fizz for all the runners as they finished the circuit. Afterwards the party carried on back in our kitchen. The celebration was in full swing when Mark stood up on one of the dining chairs to make a speech. He thanked the community for its kindness in supporting our family during those dark days; he thanked my mum for calling him a 'Twat' when he was one. He thanked our children for being more help to him than they could ever know. Looking at India he said, 'One day when you are older, you will understand what you did for me this year.'

274

Then he looked over to where I was standing next to Alison, the two of us drinking champagne out of paper cups, and he choked on his words. 'I always knew you were stubborn, but it has been amazing to watch as you have reconstructed your whole life and proved everyone wrong. You are one special woman.'

I smiled and signalled to Alison to top up my empty cup. As I took the bottle out of her hand and made sure the last dreg drained into my cup, she looked at me and said, 'The old Kate is well and truly back.'

Afterword
Reflections from a Crap Year

SOME MONTHS AFTER I returned home, Alison, Anita and I were sitting around my kitchen table, drinking Earl Grey tea, eating chocolate Hob Nobs and moaning about the men in our lives.

Suddenly the conversation turned to my recovery.

'I wonder how things would have been if Mark had had the stroke and not you?' Alison asked. 'Would he have fought so hard to get home and back on his mountain bike or would he have just accepted what the doctors said and still be in a hospital bed? I don't think my Chris would have managed so well.'

It struck me just how important a role my friends and my sheer bloody-mindedness had played in my recovery. Don't get me wrong, the doctors and nursing staff were vital keeping me alive during those crucial first hours, then helping to get those pathways in my brain working again. Even if I was too stubborn and annoyed to see it at the time, there were certain nurses who made my life in hospital bearable.

But without my friends and family, I would never have got so far, so quickly. Throughout the eight months I spent in hospital, I never once took it for granted that Anita, Alison, Jaqui and the supporting cast of Dore mums would turn up during visiting hours and spend time with me when they had so many other things to do in their busy lives.

It's funny how you never see yourself as other people do. In my mind I knew I had abnormally high expectations for myself and expected similar high standards of the people around me. But I didn't realise that my network of friends, husbands of friends and friends of friends also saw me as Kate 'the fighter'. Just days after my stroke, while I was still in a coma and my closest friends were in crisis mode, Anita's husband Bill came out with a statement that seemed so insensitive and overly optimistic that it made Mum and Mark recoil in horror. He was standing in our kitchen, looking at the canvas photo on the wall and me, Mark and the kids surfing in Cornwall, when he said: 'If I know Kate she'll be back on her feet in no time. In twelve months from now we'll all be wondering what all the fuss was about.'

Bill's comments were echoed by other villagers who only knew the old Kate and did not realise the devastating effect the stroke had had on me. If Bill had seen me at the time, just two points away from death on the 0-10 scale, with no flicker of movement, he would have been mortified by such a statement. Yet here we were almost twelve months later and he was right.

I realised that Alison had played an important part in my recovery. With no medical qualifications, except for a thirty-five-year-old Brownie badge in first aid, she gave me something that none of the medics could … emotional care, love and support. She never pitied me. She never talked down to me even when others did, especially when I was in that wheelchair. She often masked her true feelings, particularly when her own father was dying, so that she could always present a cheerful face when she saw me. She was my cry of anguish when I was in pain, my pick-me-up when I was depressed and my naughty sidekick when I needed to laugh. To hear her bluntly asking, 'Why are you being mardy?' when everyone else was tiptoeing around my feelings, was enough to lift me out of my moods. In short she was my angel in Kurt Geiger kitten heels. I firmly believe friends like Alison should be cloned and prescribed on the National Health Service for all stroke patients. I have since learnt of many others who have had strokes less severe than mine yet taken years to recover. I firmly believe I owe my life to Alison and her sidekick Anita.

Mark too was my saviour. If I had ever doubted our relationship before the stroke, it was sealed in the months afterwards. At all times Mark did what he thought was best for me and the family. That may not have always seemed like the right thing to do at the time, and sometimes he certainly made me mad. It's true we often disagreed, but the anger he caused inside me at times, unbeknown to any of us, actually fired me up and brought out the real fight in me, and that was worth more than positivity alone. He did without doubt save my life at 6.09 p.m. on Sunday February 7 2010, and rescued me from the hell that was locked-in syndrome. But crucially Mark protected me from the negative prognosis that the medics were giving him all the way through and believed in me.

On reflection I think the ten reasons I beat locked-in syndrome are:

1.   My fitness
2.   My husband, kids and mum
3.   My best friend, Alison and the other mums, Anita, Jaqui and the support network that visited continuously along with my mum

279

4.   My bloody-mindedness, refusing to take 'can't' as an answer

5.   My concentration to 'will' my limbs to move by staring at them and thinking 'Move, damn you'

6.   My disciplined therapy both with therapists and later practising alone

7.   Setting myself dates and goals

8.   My willingness to sign disclaimers and go against medical advice to follow my gut instincts

9.   Not knowing my full prognosis ever

10.   Laughter, the way Mark and my friends took the piss out of me instead of pitying me.

The happiest people don't have the best of everything, they just make the best of everything they have.

Kate Allatt, Facebook 2010.

I don't pretend to be an expert on strokes, but having been there and come out the other side with many of my faculties restored, I want to share my hard-earned words of wisdom with others.

No patient is the same, as I have always said everyone is individual but if there is one piece of advice here that can give someone lying locked in in an ICU unit somewhere in the world the hope and inspiration to fight on, then my twelve months on the road to recovery have not been in vain. These are the things that worked for me and my family.

Be positive. This can be hard when everyone around you is negative, but you have to believe in yourself and your own willpower. When life is shit, think of what inspires you. For me it was the *Rocky* theme and the image of Rocky on the steps which I kept inside my head when I needed motivation.

Set yourself real goals. No matter how small or insignificant. For me the long-term goal was to run and talk again, but it took time. Simple targets like sitting up, swallowing, holding a pen and using a computer were all positive steps on my long road to recovery.

Persevere with the communication board. The communication board is essential when you are locked in but can be frustrating. Put a sign up to explain the blinking system and try to get everyone to stick to it, there's nothing more frustrating than blinking for *no* when your carer thinks you mean *yes*. Include ready-made keywords on the board to speed up the conversations but don't second guess what the patient is trying to say, it's just bloody annoying.

Careful what you talk about. When a person is locked in, conversation can be difficult, but try to put yourself in his or her shoes. Are the eyes glazing over when you talk about certain subjects? If they are then change the topic, quickly. For me the worst thing early on was hearing about my children and what they were doing without me. The separation anxiety upset me and made me cry. I just wanted to know they were safe, nothing more. Other people may be saddened to hear about their pets or their work.

Take all the help that is available and then some. The Functional Electric Stimulation is vital and was essential to produce involuntary movements so that your brain opens up new pathways. It might feel like you're having an electric shock, but do it. The tilt table is ugly and uncomfortable but go with it. It will help your joints learn to carry your weight in readiness for standing alone. Wear foot and hand splints, they are uncomfortable and itch like hell, but if you are ever going to walk or use your hands again they are necessary to stop claw feet and shortened finger tendons.

Will your body to move. I would stare at my limbs and concentrate hard on ways to restore new pathways. This took weeks to work but I thought of the test-your-strength games at the funfair each day, and as I pushed my brain to think about movement I would imagine hitting the button with the hammer. The button was the brain signal racing along my nerves to hit the buzzer at the top. Each day those nerves got longer, until, bingo! the buzzer rang and my hand moved.

Practise every day. Remember the courage to continue counts. Days in hospital are long when you have nothing to do, so practise when you are alone and get your visitors to help you with the exercises.

Have something to look forward to. Whether it's a timetable of visitors, a TV guide with your favourite programmes or even the hope of a trip outside to the garden or the hospital shop, it will help relieve the boredom of long hours lying in bed.

Reconnect with the world. If, like me, you are computer savvy, get connected to the internet as soon as you are able to use a computer, and use Facebook and other social-network sites to communicate. This had an extremely positive impact on my mental health as I felt I was no longer trapped in hospital, but could communicate with friends all over the world at any time of the day or night. If you are locked in and not able to move, get your visitors to write a daily diary for you setting out your positive achievements. Funny letters written by friends and family are also a great way to pass the time for your visitors as they read them out, but can make the patient feel like he or she is still part of people's lives. Similarly emails and texts can make a patient feel alive and connected.

Question doctors. You don't have to accept everything they tell you because they are wearing white coats. Question them. Get bolshy if you need to. You may not win any medals for patient of the month, but it will get you to where you want to be – fit and back at home.

Prepare yourself for the way you look. Only look in a mirror when you are strong enough to meet the person looking back at you. Seeing the reflection of someone twenty years older staring back can be shocking. When you are happy with what you see, use a mirror to help practise mouth exercises.

Prove those doubters wrong! Play a game with them, set up a points system if you are really competitive. Every time you prove them wrong and achieve another unattainable goal, it's another point to you.

Know your own mind. After you have weighed up all the risks, if you think the risk is worth taking, do it.

The medics are worried about their jobs and being sued, it might be in your interests to try an alternative. You know your body. Your intuition is often right, doctors, therapists and nurses need to trust more. Be willing to sign medical disclaimers if you are going against medical advice but have a gut instinct you are right.

Don't put limits on your recovery and time-frame, any improvement is possible at any time if you can keep your mind optimistic and strong, however hard that is.

Channel your anger. If doctors or your loved ones make you angry by failing to move at your pace, don't get angry, get active. They may not even realise you're upset, so convert your anger into a 'sod you, I will do it,' attitude and do it. It worked for me, even though my doctors, nurses and friends didn't deliberately set out to make me angry!

Finally…

Don't spend your days dreaming, get working. Life's too short! And don't ignore headaches.

Acknowledgements

With the first anniversary gone, I thought it was appropriate to thank a few people in this book. My mum who did what only mums do best – for the first time in a long time, I was your baby. Alison French, best friend and 'partner in crime', who never took a vow to care for me, like you would in marriages, but her daftness, support, non-judgmental friendship and non-pitying approach, were remarkable. Her instinct, support and selflessness, regardless of her terrible own bad year, was invaluable. Anita Hine and Jaqui Perryer, my long-suffering running pals, who stood by me and rallied so much, being both practical and motherly. To all the staff at the ICU who kept me alive and the therapists, especially Emma who treated me like one of the girls and Oliver, with the sarcastic humour, who kept me going and indulged me in my love of The Smiths.

Amy, Sharon, Sarah and Kerry, your coarse sense of humour and laughs got me through. To my stepdad, Dave, my sister Abi and my in-laws Ann and Kev – 'how dare you leave your slippers under the stairs!' To Jo for keeping me manicured throughout! To Ali for being a surrogate mum and Rob for being eye candy for the nurses! To Anna's infamous fish pie! To all the church ladies who cooked for Mark and my kids in my absence. To Michael, my personal trainer, along with Alister, from Esporta Health & Fitness, who helped me keep on schedule and gave me a second chance of life. To Alison Stokes, who pieced my immense volume of content together into a readable format and also for helping me pass on my legacy to my kids and helping me to give help and real hope to other locked-in syndrome sufferers, their families and friends. To Hazel at Accent Press, if you had not found me on Facebook I would never have had the opportunity to publish my story. To John at SM4B who created my Facebook page and Allan and Annie who both created my fabulous logo for my Fighting Strokes charity. To Anne Marie for her kindness and prayers and to Lise from next door who literally saved my life. To Riasca printers and the Rotary Club of Southport Links. To Lindsay and Sue at the Co-op, who showed my kids such warmth. To Sue Hopkinson and Dore Primary School. To Lisa for her amazing lemon ginger cake! Especially the mums who bought me such lovely Clarins creams in the ICU. To the Derbyshire Freemasons for their ongoing support and fund-raising. To the girlies in my book group, hope you give this a kind review! To everyone who supported my bike ride and fundraising event at Derwent Reservoir, thanks so much. To my first best mate Donna, thanks for being back so much and for my holiday to Disney! To my 'fans' on Facebook and Twitter who followed me and gave me the strength to keep fighting. To the mountain-bike husbands, Chris, James, Bill, Andy, Simon, Adrian and Gary, thanks for being there to listen to Mark's jokes and sick sense of humour! To Mark for proving how much he loved me, he really did honour his wedding vows and was there, often with the unenviable job of making such tough decisions. To my kids who are, and have been, so resilient through all this, even though their honeymoon period of good behaviour is over!

I hope this book raises awareness, real hope and gives practical help and advice to other survivors of locked-in syndrome and younger stroke survivors. Whoever said the community is dead? I have lived all over the world and I can assure you that I wouldn't want to live anywhere else but Dore.

Heartfelt thanks to you all.

Kate

Appendix
Recently Affected by Locked-in Syndrome? My Tips

First establish with patients:
- If they understand yes/no questions and are therefore not brain damaged.

Then establish,
- One blink or look down for no
- Two blinks or look up for yes
- Blank stare if patient doesn't know the answer

- Are you in pain?
- Are you comfortable?
- Are you hot?
- Are you cold?
- Do you get turned enough?
- Do you understand why your foot and hand splints are so important?
- Do you want some headphones to listen to music?
- Would you prefer your music via some speakers?
- Is there any music you really don't like?
- If you have a breathing tube, are you comfortable?
- Do you get cramp?
- If so, can we ease this?
- Can you give us a sign for right leg or left leg?

- If you have a tracheotomy, does it pop off?
- Does that frighten you?
- Are you sleeping at night?
- Are you sleeping in the day?
- Do you want sleeping pills?
- Do you hear things that have frightened you?
- Do you want to see your kids?
- Do you want to hear what they are doing, other than to know they are safe?
- Have they explained what happened to you?
- Have they explained your treatment plans?
- Do you know how important it is to start fighting this to get back to your old life asap?

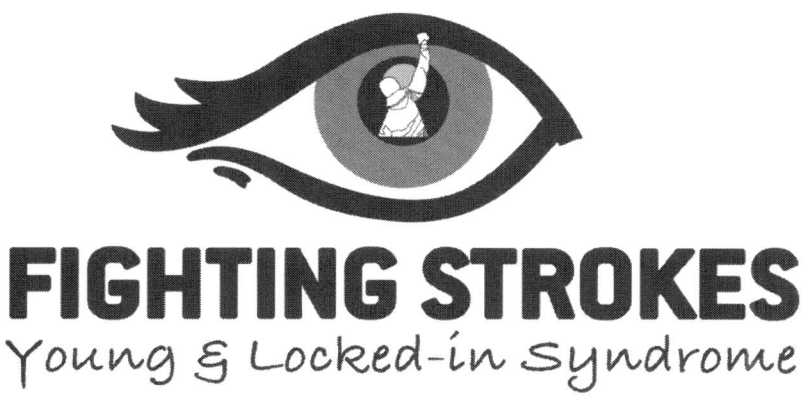

FIGHTING STROKES
Young & Locked-in Syndrome

'Empower & inspire those affected by all strokes,
including Locked in Syndrome,
who are under 60 years of age'

Aims

- Raise awareness.
- Inform care-givers and health professional working with survivors.
- Provide support for family and friends.
- Provide patient support.

http://www.fightingstrokes.org

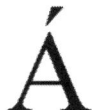

Proudly published by Accent Press

www.accentpress.co.uk

Printed in Poland
by Amazon Fulfillment
Poland Sp. z o.o., Wrocław

50873934R00176